THE HERBAL FERTILITY HANDBOOK

Natural Strategies to
**INCREASE YOUR CHANCES
of GETTING PREGNANT**

LIANE MOCCIA, RH (AHG)

Storey Publishing

The mission of Storey Publishing is to serve our customers by publishing practical information that encourages personal independence in harmony with the environment.

EDITED BY Carleen Madigan and Sarah Guare Slattery
ART DIRECTION AND BOOK DESIGN BY Erin Dawson
TEXT PRODUCTION BY Jennifer Jepson Smith

COVER PHOTOGRAPHY BY Mars Vilaubi © Storey Publishing and Dragonfly Photography (author)
FOOD STYLING BY Sophie Gerry
ILLUSTRATIONS BY © BlueRingMedia/Shutterstock.com, 20; Isometrik, Kaldari; Begoon; Marnanel/
CC BY-SA 3.0/Wikimedia Commons, 15, 35; © Natalia Zelenina/Shutterstock.com, 57;
© Peter Hermes Furian/Shutterstock.com, 22

This publication is intended to provide educational information for the reader on the covered subject. It is not intended to take the place of personalized medical counseling, diagnosis, and treatment from a trained health professional. Please consult a physician or other health professional if needed.

Storey Publishing
210 MASS MoCA Way
North Adams, MA 01247
storey.com

Storey Publishing is an imprint of Workman Publishing, a division of Hachette Book Group, Inc., 1290 Avenue of the Americas, New York, NY 10104. The Storey Publishing name and logo are registered trademarks of Hachette Book Group, Inc.

ISBNs: 978-1-63586-873-9 (paperback);
978-1-63586-874-6 (ebook)

Printed in the United States by Versa Press on paper from responsible sources
10 9 8 7 6 5 4 3 2 1

VER

Library of Congress Cataloging-in-Publication Data on file

To my daughters:
Our journey brought me here.
Without it, my work simply
wouldn't exist.

Contents

INTRODUCTION

Planting the Seeds of Fertility

No matter where you are on your journey to parenthood—just getting started, somewhere in the middle, wondering why this is taking so long, or deep into the 1-year wait (the time period most doctors recommend trying on your own), a holistic approach to fertility can support you and your goal of getting pregnant, and, as an added bonus, boost your overall wellness.

The prep work for starting a family is a bit like gardening. It involves a lot more than picking out nursery colors and debating baby names. Think of it like this: When you're envisioning a bountiful harvest of fresh veggies, you don't simply close your eyes and poof, tomatoes and carrots are magically ready for picking. It requires thoughtful planning—selecting a sunny spot, clearing out weeds, enriching the soil, planting top-notch seeds, and faithfully watering. With time, care, and patience your garden will flourish. Similarly, taking the time to prep your bodies before pregnancy can significantly impact both your and your partner's fertility, the health of the pregnancy, and, ultimately, your baby's health.

Anyone ready to begin building their family will benefit from a holistic view of their fertility, which includes supporting both egg and sperm health. Too often the burden of trying to conceive falls on the person who ovulates. Time, money, and hours of endlessly searching "how to improve fertility" can be wasted if both aspects are not considered.

Holistic Strategies to Help You Conceive

Centuries of herbal medicine combined with decades of scientific research have confirmed that you absolutely can improve your chances of getting pregnant by incorporating herbs, making changes to your diet, modifying certain aspects of your lifestyle, and limiting exposure to toxins in your environment. In my role as an herbalist specializing in fertility and preconception planning, I've witnessed the remarkable potential of integrating herbs and lifestyle modifications to promote fertility, support well-being, and restore balance to our bodies.

Certain herbs stand out as nutritional powerhouses, fostering general health, fertility, and virility, while others are tailored to address specific health challenges. But herbs aren't the whole story when it comes to a holistic fertility plan. Herbs aren't a panacea; they aren't a replacement for managing stress, getting good sleep, and eating well. That's why this book offers a fully holistic approach to support all aspects of your fertility.

The goal of this book is to provide simple, holistic, and evidence-based strategies to help improve your chances of getting pregnant. These strategies include nutrition, herbs, supplements, environmental exposures, and lifestyle factors such as sleep, stress, movement, and more. Your relationship status, conception method, previous infertility diagnosis, or where you are in the process does not play a role here. Whether you are in a partnered relationship, single and using an egg or sperm donor, or in a same-sex partnership; just starting to try for a baby or have been trying for a few months or years; conceiving naturally or going through assisted reproductive technologies, it really doesn't matter. The point is that taking steps to support your fertility will help improve your chances of getting pregnant. Period.

The approach I take in my practice is to help people control the things they can, allowing them to worry less about those they can't. This same philosophy is true for *The Herbal Fertility Handbook*.

While the focus of this book is to improve your chances of getting pregnant, the strategies are all backed by scientific research, can be easily incorporated into your daily life, and will help support your overall health, wellness, and fertility. In addition to being a registered herbalist who helps clients get pregnant and educates others on the herbal effect on fertility, I've also been in your shoes. I've personally navigated the emotions of frustration, confusion, disappointment, fear, and even anger when trying to become pregnant.

My Pregnancy Journey

My own struggle with infertility is what started me down the path toward becoming an herbalist. My husband and I never expected to have a hard time getting pregnant. I was so frustrated (and scared) during that first year of trying that I actually lied to my doctor. I am not proud to admit this, but it's true. After 8 months of trying I didn't want to just "try for 1 year" before investigating other options. So I lied to my obstetrician and said we'd been trying to conceive for a full 12 months. Spoiler alert: She was on to me and encouraged me to keep going and wait out the full year before moving on to any fertility testing.

Don't get me wrong, I respected my doctor, but I was desperate. I was willing to do anything. I went headfirst down the rabbit hole of research, scouring the internet and every book I could find. This is when I first discovered the potential for herbal remedies.

Looking back, I couldn't understand why there weren't more options for us during that first year. Why didn't anyone ask about our diet, check for certain vitamin deficiencies or hormone imbalances, or talk to us about environmental exposures? After being told our sperm parameters were "within normal limits," sperm health was never discussed again. Finally, after being diagnosed with diminished ovarian reserve and having three intrauterine insemination (IUI) and four in vitro fertilization (IVF) cycles, we conceived our twins.

Knowing what I know now, the reality is that we could have done more . . . a lot more. I have seen the difference herbs and nutrition can make. Knowing there was more we could have done to support our fertility fueled my passion to help others, so I went back to school, became a registered herbalist, and completed a mentorship with a renowned naturopathic fertility doctor in Boston. Now I help people optimize their fertility through herbs, nutrition, and lifestyle changes. Having a clear plan can take so much pressure off you when you are trying to conceive.

Think of the recommendations in this book as an à la carte menu. I invite you to start slow, try a few things that sound reasonable and doable in your current situation, and then build up over time. Don't feel like you need to do everything all at once. Simple, small changes will have an impact.

My hope is that reading this book will empower you to take an active role in your fertility, to look at the whole picture (including both partners if there are two), destigmatize and normalize conversations around both the egg and the sperm factors, and provide simple, evidence-based strategies to support overall health and fertility.

You are not alone in this journey.

CHAPTER 1

FERTILITY 101

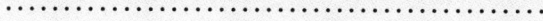

···

Common Thoughts and Misconceptions

Sperm meets egg and makes an embryo—
it's a simple formula that we all learned in high school
biology. Well, it's not actually quite that easy.

Your Chances of Getting Pregnant

For a healthy, ovulating person in their 20s or early 30s, the chance of getting pregnant is about 25–30 percent in any single menstrual cycle. The percentage starts to decline in a person's early 30s, and by age 40 the chance drops to less than 10 percent per cycle. But remember, these statistics are based on averages and don't necessarily represent *your* actual chances. The strategies in this book are meant to help you beat the "average" and increase your individual odds of getting pregnant.

The Interminable 1-Year Wait

Technically speaking, infertility is defined as not getting pregnant after at least 12 months of regular, unprotected sexual intercourse. Current guidelines follow suit, indicating that people under 35 years of age try for 12 months before being referred to a specialist for a fertility evaluation (or 6 months if you are over 35 years old). Eight to 12.5 percent of couples worldwide are considered to have infertility issues.[1] Maybe you don't fall into this percentage of people with an official diagnosis of infertility, but you have been trying to conceive and things are taking longer than you'd hoped.

This period of time is often referred to as the "1-year wait" and can be filled with anxiety, frustration, and a lot of uncertainty. Couples feel like each month is an eternity, and they want to do more (something, anything!) to shorten the time it takes to get pregnant or fast-track a fertility evaluation. Trust me, I've been there.

These feelings of unease exist in the months before the "magical" 1-year timeline has been reached. You and your partner don't fall into a particular statistics bucket, and therefore reside in a sort of fertility limbo, with no answers or solutions in sight. The decision you've made to start a family is a journey, and there will be many twists and turns and detours along the way. However, knowing that you are not alone can be a huge comfort.

The science behind getting and staying pregnant shows that it's rather miraculous it happens at all, but you can certainly increase your chances of getting pregnant by utilizing some of the strategies discussed in this book to increase your fertility. Simple, evidence-based strategies that include using certain herbs, nutrients, and supplements; reducing environmental exposures; and making lifestyle changes can help improve sperm and egg health, and ultimately can increase your odds of becoming pregnant.

How Conception Really Happens

The process of natural conception begins with ejaculation, in which millions of sperm are released in a fluid called semen. The sperm travel, propelled by their tail and assisted by waves of fluid inside the uterus, from the vagina, through the cervix, to the uterus and fallopian tubes where they (hopefully!) meet the egg. It's a race to the top of the reproductive tract, and the winner gets the egg.

The trick is overcoming the many obstacles encountered along the way. For example, sperm don't always swim in the right direction (or at all), the acidity of the vagina and cervical mucus has to be just right, and then there's the potential of taking a wrong turn and going to the wrong (i.e., eggless) fallopian tube. If all of this goes well and the sperm reaches the correct fallopian tube, some will bind to its surface leaving only a few to continue on to meet an egg. If there's no egg there yet, that's okay—sperm can live in the fallopian tubes for up to 5 days, whereas an egg only lives for about 24 hours. So it's better for the sperm to arrive early and wait for the ovulated egg to arrive.

The Process of Fertilization

When everything is in alignment and a sperm connects with an egg, it goes through a process called the acrosome reaction. After the sperm's membrane binds to the egg's outer membrane, the contents of the sperm's acrosome—the "cap" on the top of the sperm's pointed head—are exposed. The enzymes within the acrosome begin to dissolve the tough outer layers of the egg and the tail begins to "beat" faster so the head of the sperm can sink into the egg. Many sperm may start this process by fusing to the outside of the egg, but once a single sperm enters the egg's interior, the egg's membrane hardens, preventing other sperm from penetrating. At this point, the sperm's nucleus, which carries all of the DNA, floats into the egg's interior fluid, called cytoplasm. This is the moment of fertilization. There are still uncertainties to overcome before this fertilized egg becomes an embryo, but fertilization is where it all begins.

The quality of the egg also influences the likelihood of fertilization. Eggs that have abnormal DNA (known as aneuploidy) either fail to fertilize or fertilize but end in miscarriage or, if carried to term, can result in genetic disorders for the baby. See Chapter 2 for more on this.

From Zygote to Implantation

When a sperm and an egg combine, they each contribute 23 chromosomes, resulting in a new organism called a zygote, with 46 chromosomes. These influence hundreds of characteristics, including skin tone, hair texture, dimples, height, and eye color, which are determined instantly and are a result of joining together both sets of chromosomes.

The resulting zygote moves down the fallopian tube, dividing several times. Roughly a week after the sperm has fertilized the egg, the zygote will have traveled to the uterus and will be a growing cluster of about 100 cells. This is called a blastocyst.

If all goes well, the blastocyst attaches itself to the lining of the uterus (the endometrium). This attachment process is called implantation. However, just because conception occurs doesn't mean implantation will. Both the uterus's ability to accept the embryo and the embryo's health are key for the implantation process. Sometimes implantation doesn't happen or the embryo stops developing. In these cases, the blastocyst is passed with the next menstrual period. This is often referred to as a chemical pregnancy or early miscarriage that happens within the first 5 weeks of pregnancy, so early that it often goes undetected.

It is truly the survival of the fittest—the general consensus is that this arduous journey is nature's way of weeding out the weaker sperm and eggs, thereby creating an environment to produce a stronger, healthier baby.

On average, even under perfectly timed conditions, with good swimmers who know their directions, a healthy egg, normal DNA, and receptive uterine lining, conception happens only 25–30 percent of the time. It's kind of a miracle pregnancy ever occurs at all.

Using certain herbs, nutrients, and supplements; reducing environmental exposures; and making lifestyle changes can help improve sperm and egg health, and ultimately can increase your odds of becoming pregnant.

CHAPTER 2

WHY
EGG
QUALITY
MATTERS

....

Demystifying the Factors That Influence Egg Health and Fertility

The quality of an egg plays a crucial role in a person's fertility, and over time, both the quantity and quality of a person's eggs naturally decline. However, this fact tells only part of the story.

Can We Actually Improve Egg Quality?

When I first met Emily, she and her partner had been trying to conceive for almost a year. She was 34 years old and beginning to worry that age was playing a role in how long it was taking them to get pregnant. She started searching "how to improve fertility" online, but after endless scrolling and several rabbit holes later, she was only confused and overwhelmed by the long list of things that may (or may not) be right for her. On top of that, friends eagerly gave their input and shared what worked for them. It felt like everyone around her was sharing pregnancy announcements and new baby photos.

Disheartened, Emily made an appointment with her obstetrician. Armed with her list of advice, research, supplements, natural remedies, lifestyle adjustments, and wives' tales, she felt confident her doctor could help her sort through everything and come up with a plan. Her doctor took one look at her list and said, "Emily, you were born with all of your eggs, and those eggs have been exposed to damage and the natural process of aging over your lifetime. Do you really think taking a few supplements will reverse 30 years? Save your money, take a prenatal multivitamin, and just keep trying."

Needless to say, Emily left feeling discouraged, sad, and frustrated. Unfortunately, this advice is given out more often than you might think, but it is an oversimplification and ignores what we (the scientific community) know about egg maturation in the 4 months before ovulation.

To address Emily's situation: Can we turn back time and completely reverse aging and possible damage done to our eggs? No. But we can most certainly support our eggs to give them their best chance. The changes we make today will affect the egg that is ovulated approximately 4 months from now. In this chapter, I cover how an egg develops and matures and how to support the process for the best chance of improving egg quality.

Let's dig deeper into the science behind egg development and maturation. Follow along with Emily's journey throughout the book to see what we did to support her fertility.

The Science Behind Egg Quality

You may think "an egg is an egg," but the truth is that not all eggs are created equal. Individuals with ovaries will ovulate hundreds of eggs over their lifetime, but when it comes to conceiving, the quality of these eggs matters. This is where factors like age, ovulation cycles, lifestyle, and diet come into play. Many people are surprised to learn there is a 4-month window before an egg ovulates when it undergoes significant changes and maturation. This window is the time when we can have the biggest impact on the egg's quality.

Understanding the Egg

Let's start by better understanding the egg and what needs to happen in order to get pregnant. The human egg is unlike any other cell in the body. It stops halfway through its growth cycle and remains in a state of suspended animation for years until it's ready to ovulate. A few months prior to ovulation, the egg "wakes up" from this state of hibernation and undergoes a process of growth and maturation.

This process is incredibly energy- and nutrient-intensive on the body. The quality of the ovulating egg is greatly influenced by external exposure during the months before ovulation, which means there is an opportunity to positively affect egg quality through your choice of diet, herbs, and supplements; reducing environmental exposures; and addressing lifestyle factors such as sleep, stress, and movement.

EGG MYTHS . . . BUSTED

MYTH: I'm young so my eggs are all good!

FACT: People under age 35 are less likely to have issues with egg quality, but age is still a factor. Egg quality will affect how long it takes to become pregnant and can increase the risk of miscarriage.

Research shows that 25 percent of the eggs a person under age 35 ovulates are chromosomally abnormal and unlikely to result in a pregnancy or birth.[1] Let's boil that statistic down and see what this means for the average, healthy, regularly ovulating person over the course of a year. If everything is working properly and timed perfectly, instead of 12 opportunities to conceive in a year, there may actually be only 9.

MYTH: There's nothing I can do to improve my egg quality.

FACT: The 4-month window before an egg ovulates gives every ovulating person the opportunity to support egg development by providing everything the egg needs to be its healthiest.

Age Makes a Difference

The truth is that the age of the ovulating person has a big impact on pregnancy success rates. Egg quantity declines as we age, and the percentage of chromosomally abnormal eggs ovulated each month increases. At some point, an ovulating individual may be too old to use their own eggs to achieve a pregnancy (that age will vary for every person and can be influenced by genetics and lifestyle), and if they have gone through menopause, they can't use their own eggs to become pregnant. For people over age 40, more than half of the eggs ovulated may be chromosomally abnormal. These are the statistics, but this doesn't have to be your reality.

The good news is that the quality of a person's eggs does not need to be in steady, linear decline from early adulthood until menopause. Egg quality can vary from month to month, influenced by the resources available to the egg and the external environmental exposures. What does this mean? You absolutely have the ability to improve the health of every cell in your body, including the cells in ovaries.

Egg Development 101

The process of egg production starts before a person is even born. Yes, you read that correctly! It begins during the first trimester of the mother's pregnancy. Babies with ovaries are born with all of the eggs (called oocytes) they will ever have. (See Are People Really Born with All Their Eggs? on page 12.) These oocytes lie dormant in the ovaries until puberty, when a handful start the maturation process resulting in only one egg ovulating approximately every month. The number of oocytes a person has is in a constant state of decline from one to two million at birth, to approximately 200,000 at puberty, to about one thousand or fewer remaining at menopause.

Four Months from Dormancy to Ovulation

The journey of an egg from its dormant state to ovulation takes about 4 months and starts with an initial pool of 6 to 15 eggs (called primordial oocytes). Each primordial oocyte develops within its own sac, called a follicle. As the follicles grow, they receive signals from the body's hormones, such as follicle-stimulating hormone (FSH), that give instructions on how and when to grow.

The follicles continue to develop and produce increasing amounts of the estrogen hormone. Eventually, one becomes the dominant follicle: It grows faster and becomes the most advanced. This dominant follicle will eventually release a mature egg during ovulation. The other follicles that were not selected as the dominant one will shrink and be reabsorbed by the body. Roughly 99 percent of the follicles in the ovary will not make it to ovulation.

Just prior to ovulation, a surge of luteinizing hormone (LH) triggers the oocyte to restart its cell development, and important chromosomal reorganization occurs. If things go wrong during this stage, the oocyte ends up with an extra or missing copy of a chromosome, resulting in a chromosomally abnormal egg that is unlikely to survive to pregnancy or birth. If everything goes right, a chromosomally normal egg develops, which has a better chance of survival.

The entire process relies on precise hormonal regulation and a rich supply of nutrients and antioxidants, and is incredibly energy-intensive. Environmental factors, lifestyle, and genetics all contribute to the success or failure of developing and ovulating a healthy egg.

When someone is trying to conceive, there's a lot of focus on ovulation: When will it happen, did it happen, is it regular and predictable, did intercourse occur in time? In reality, the months leading up to ovulation are where you can make the biggest impact.

The underlying message is supporting egg quality in the months leading up to ovulation can impact the quality of the ovulated egg and increase the percentage of good quality eggs so they will have a better chance of getting fertilized, implanting, and developing into a healthy baby.

ARE PEOPLE REALLY BORN
WITH ALL THEIR EGGS?

The accepted belief that all ovulating individuals are born with a fixed number of eggs that gradually diminish over their lifetime came into question in 2004 when an animal study suggested the presence of special cells in mouse ovaries that could generate new eggs. This discovery sparked significant controversy and has since led to extensive research and debate. Despite ongoing studies, definitive evidence is still lacking to confirm the existence of these cells, called oocyte-stem cells. The scientific community holds passionately diverse opinions on this topic. While preliminary studies have shown promising results regarding the existence of these cells and their ability to create new eggs, many questions remain unanswered. There is no evidence at this time that would lead to a change in clinical treatment.[2]

Antioxidants and Egg Quality

Studies on infertility have found that oxidative stress may be one of the reasons some couples struggle to conceive. But what exactly does that mean?

Oxidative stress happens when there's an imbalance between antioxidants and free radicals. Free radicals can cause damage to our DNA, proteins, and lipids, wreaking havoc on all cells, including the eggs and sperm.

Free radicals are produced naturally in our bodies during various processes. They can also come from external sources like radiation, pollution, and smoking. Among these free radicals, there is a specific group called reactive oxygen species (ROS), which contain oxygen. Oxidative stress occurs when there's an increase in ROS because the cells don't have enough antioxidants to neutralize them. These oxidizing substances play important roles in our bodies' normal functions and overall health, including fertility.

Simply put, oxidative stress can negatively affect the development of eggs, the functioning of the ovaries, and the chances of getting pregnant. As you'll see in Chapter 3, oxidative stress can also negatively impact sperm health.

The good news is the herbs, nutrients, supplements, and lifestyle recommendations throughout this book will help support a balance between antioxidants and free radicals.

A Closer Look at the Menstrual Cycle

One of my biggest pet peeves is the misinformation that is spread about the menstrual cycle. Just like every person is unique, so, too, is their cycle. In general, the whole process is way more complex than you might think and is definitely more than just a monthly bleed.

So why is a menstrual cycle so important to understand? Because it can inform the timing of intercourse and is also a vital sign, just like temperature or blood pressure, providing insight and information regarding general health and fertility. Understanding the phases and hormones involved is a crucial part of a holistic fertility plan.

The menstrual cycle involves multiple organs that interact and coordinate with each other in a precise manner. The brain, ovaries, and uterus are like dance partners, moving together in a choreographed routine. This dance is a series of events where hormones and feedback loops play a key role. It's a delicate process of coordination and communication that keeps everything working together.

MENSTRUAL CYCLE MYTHS . . . BUSTED

MYTH: The average menstrual cycle is 28 days.
FACT: Only 13 percent of cycles are 28 days long.[3] Most range between 21 and 35 days long; a healthy cycle is between 24 and 38 days.

MYTH: Ovulation occurs on day 14.
FACT: Not always—as menstrual cycles vary in length, so does the timing of ovulation.

MYTH: Getting a period means you definitely ovulated that month.
FACT: Unfortunately, no. An individual can still have a period even if they're not ovulating. (Technically, it's not a period, but practically, they're still dealing with bleeding.)

Phases of Menstruation

A healthy menstrual cycle ranges between 24 and 38 days. Starting with the first full day of a period (also called cycle day 1), the ovaries communicate with the brain to develop and release an egg for fertilization while the uterus sheds its lining and then rebuilds to prepare for pregnancy. At a high level, the menstrual cycle is broken down into the following phases:

The follicular phase. During this phase—which begins on the first day of menstruation and goes approximately through mid-cycle—the brain (specifically the hypothalamus and pituitary gland) communicates with the ovaries by releasing FSH, which signals the ovaries to grow and mature a group of follicles. These follicles contain eggs, and as they develop, one becomes the dominant follicle that will ovulate a mature egg. As the follicles mature, they release estrogen, the dominant hormone in this phase. Estrogen thickens the uterine lining after it was shed during menstruation, creating an ideal environment for embryo implantation, and stimulates the cervix to produce cervical fluid that helps sperm swim more easily and reach the egg for fertilization.

Ovulation. This happens approximately mid-cycle. The estrogen rise that occurs as the dominant follicle develops triggers the brain to switch from secreting FSH to secreting LH. LH rapidly increases until it reaches a surge, which is necessary to trigger ovulation. (Side note: This surge is what home ovulation predictor kits detect.) Right before the LH surge, estrogen levels fall. This abrupt hormonal shift triggers ovulation, which is the release of the egg from the ovary. The egg is then swept up and enters the fallopian tube, where it will survive for about 24 hours. Because sperm can survive for several days, the most fertile period is about 5 days before ovulation until 1 to 2 days after ovulation.

The luteal phase. This is from ovulation until the first day of bleeding. After ovulation, the empty follicle transforms into a temporary structure called the corpus luteum. The corpus luteum produces estrogen and progesterone, with progesterone being the dominant hormone in this phase. Progesterone's main job is to support the uterine lining for a possible pregnancy.

If fertilization occurs, the embryo signals the corpus luteum to keep producing progesterone until the placenta can take over. If fertilization doesn't occur, the corpus luteum stops producing progesterone, leading to menstruation. The luteal phase should last at least 11 days so there is enough time for the embryo to implant before the uterine lining is shed. The drop in progesterone signals the brain to restart the cycle, and the whole process begins again.

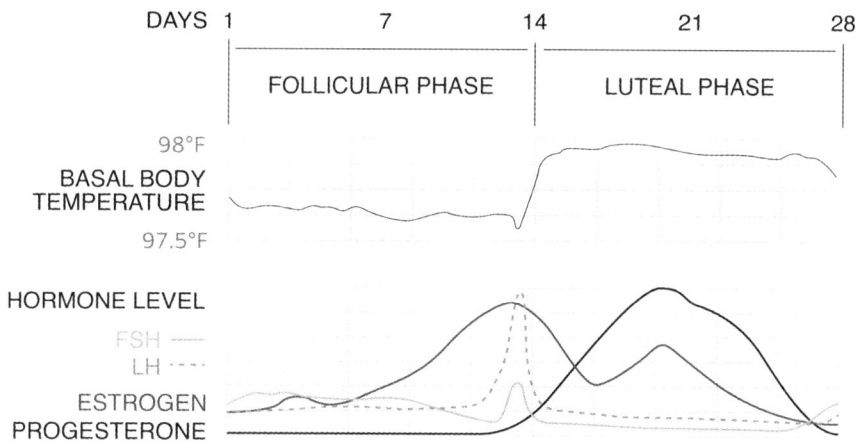

A well-balanced hormone communication between the brain and ovaries, known as the hypothalamic-pituitary-ovarian (HPO) axis, is essential for a healthy cycle. The hormones involved in this intricate dance help develop healthy follicles, trigger ovulation, and support the early stages of pregnancy. In Chapter 5, I cover the testing and blood work that is often ordered to evaluate the hormones involved in this process. In Chapter 11, I delve into common conditions that can impact fertility, including situations where the HPO axis encounters difficulties.

MYTHS ABOUT HOW THE PILL
AFFECTS FERTILITY . . . BUSTED

When it comes to birth control pills, there are misconceptions regarding their impact on future fertility. Let's address the top two myths.

MYTH: Being on the pill makes it harder to get pregnant when you stop taking it.
FACT: Studies show that fertility typically returns to normal within three menstrual cycles after stopping oral contraceptives. After a year, former pill users have similar pregnancy rates to those who used non-hormonal methods.

MYTH: The pill *regulates* the menstrual cycle.
FACT: The pill *suppresses* the menstrual cycle by interrupting signals from the brain to prevent ovulation; or altering the uterine lining, making it less receptive to implantation; or thickening cervical fluid to impede sperm movement. However, it may mask underlying fertility-affecting conditions, which can resurface once pill usage stops. These conditions, not the pill itself, may impact fertility. Chapter 11 explores common conditions affecting fertility.

The bottom line is this: Don't worry that past pill use is getting in the way of getting pregnant now.

CHAPTER 3

WHY
SPERM
QUALITY
MATTERS

··

It's Time to Take the Burden
Solely off the Eggs

It takes two to tango, as the old adage goes. Nothing could be more true when it comes to trying to get pregnant. Seems obvious, right? You need both a sperm and an egg before any conception can even start to happen. It is, quite simply, the way science and nature work. You *cannot* have one without the other. So why is it that I often hear a more one-sided story?

It Takes Two to Get Pregnant

Over coffee, a friend shared that her sister was "unable to get pregnant." She and her partner had been trying to get pregnant without success. They had no formal workup, no diagnosis, and no reason to believe there was something "wrong" with her sister.

Too often we hear "she" was unable to get pregnant instead of "she and her partner have not been able to get pregnant." Aren't there two people involved in this process? The answer is yes.

Even though it feels like most conversations focus on ovulation, egg quality, or uterine health, that is because society tends to place the burden of trying to conceive solely on the ovulating partner. The truth is that sperm health matters, too. Fifty percent of all infertility cases have sperm-related factors, and 20 percent of infertility cases are *solely* the result of sperm factors.

If you as a couple or individual fall into the 50 percent whose sperm health is contributing to infertility (or subfertility, which is any form of reduced fertility with prolonged time to pregnancy), then you could be wasting time and money addressing only part of the fertility equation.

Fifty percent of all infertility cases have sperm-related factors, and 20 percent of infertility cases are *solely* the result of sperm factors.

Sperm Production and Anatomy

It takes 64 days for the testes to create new sperm, a process that is called spermatogenesis. During this time, environmental factors, nutrients, and lifestyle choices can impact the process and affect the quality of the sperm. A new spermatogenesis cycle starts approximately every 16 days. Because it takes a couple of months for a complete cycle of spermatogenesis, any changes a person starts today will affect the sperm that is released approximately 2 months later.

The Science Behind Testosterone and Sperm

Testosterone is the primary hormone involved in sperm production and is a critical ingredient in making a baby as well as in supporting healthy sperm, sex drive, and erectile function; maintaining muscle strength and mass; and promoting bone density. In general, maintaining normal concentrations of testosterone promotes spermatogenesis, whereas low levels of testosterone can lead to infertility.

THE BRAIN–TESTES FEEDBACK LOOP

Similar to how the brain and the ovaries are in constant communication to develop and ovulate an egg, testosterone and sperm production are precisely regulated by a feedback loop between the brain and the testes.

The hypothalamus is the region in the brain that monitors the body's level of testosterone and produces gonadotropin-releasing hormone (GnRH) when it detects low levels. GnRH travels to the anterior pituitary gland, where it stimulates the release of two important hormones: FSH and LH. FSH and LH modulate testosterone production and spermatogenesis from specific cells in the testes. High levels of testosterone signal the hypothalamus to reduce the production and release of GnRH, which, in turn, reduces the secretion of FSH and LH from the pituitary gland. The decrease in FSH and LH levels subsequently reduces the stimulation of the testes, leading to a decrease in testosterone production. The brain–testes feedback loop helps both maintain testosterone levels within a certain range and keep hormone levels in balance.

The regulation of testosterone and other hormones in the body is critical for maintaining healthy sperm production and overall hormonal balance. The feedback system ensures that hormone levels remain within a narrow range, preventing excessive or deficient hormone production. Anything that disrupts this feedback loop can decrease production of testosterone and sperm. For example, certain medications, stress, overexercising, poor nutrition, lack of sleep, and obesity can all negatively affect the delicate balance and contribute to decreased sperm.

Natural strategies, including herbs, nutrition, and lifestyle changes, will help support the body's ability to make testosterone and sperm. We cover these strategies in depth throughout this book.

A DROP IN TESTOSTERONE

Testosterone levels have declined across the world's population, with individuals today having lower levels than those of the same age a generation ago. This decline is accelerating, fueled by factors like poor diet, chronic stress, inactivity, and environmental toxins.

STEP AWAY FROM TESTOSTERONE
REPLACEMENT THERAPY

A common misconception is that if naturally occurring testosterone is good for sperm, then supplementing with testosterone will improve sperm and fertility. In truth, supplementing with testosterone shuts down the body's ability to produce its own naturally.

In order for sperm production to occur, there must be a high concentration of testosterone in the testicles, which only happens when the testosterone is made in the testicles, as opposed to when it is circulating in the bloodstream.

When a person uses testosterone replacement therapy, the excess testosterone circulating in the blood sends a signal to the brain that no additional testosterone is needed. The pituitary then begins decreasing production of LH and FSH, shutting down production of testosterone and sperm in the testes.

It's common for people on testosterone replacement therapy to experience low or zero sperm count. In most cases, the effects can be reversed by stopping the testosterone supplement and waiting for internal testosterone levels to rise again. This process can take anywhere from a few weeks to a few years, and can occasionally result in permanent infertility.

ANATOMY OF SPERM

Sperm cells are approximately 0.05 millimeters long and are made up of three distinct parts.

- The head, which contains the tightly packed genetic information (DNA) plus the acrosomal vesicle (a structure at the tip of the sperm that helps the sperm penetrate the egg)

- The midpiece, which contains cells to produce energy used to power the sperm's movement

- The tail, which helps the sperm swim toward the egg

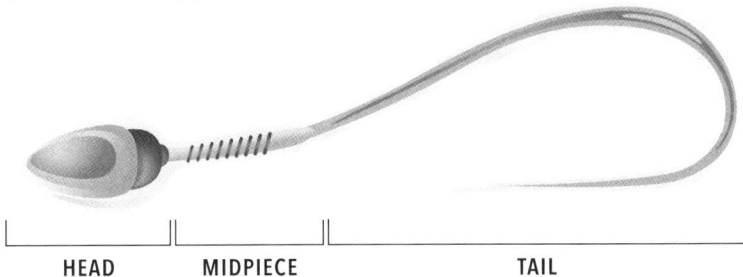

HEAD   MIDPIECE   TAIL

Creating Healthy Sperm Anatomy

Healthy sperm anatomy is critical to a sperm's ability to travel and penetrate an egg. There's a lot that goes into creating this healthy environment, including the right temperature and adequate amounts of nutrients, including vitamins, minerals, and antioxidants.

COOL TEMPERATURES KEEP SPERM ALIVE

Ever wonder why testicles hang low? Cooler temperatures are important for spermatogenesis, which is why the testicles descend from the body. This keeps them about 4°F (2°C) cooler than the usual body temperature of 98.6°F (37°C).

HEAT KILLS: HOW TO PROTECT SPERM

Anything that increases the temperature of the testicles, even for a relatively short period of time, can hurt sperm. Avoid the following to give sperm their best chance.

- Tight-fitting underwear and pants

- Hot tubs and long baths

- Saunas

- Placing a laptop on your lap for an extended period of time

- Long spin classes or bike rides

- Heated car seats

- Sitting for prolonged periods of time

ANTIOXIDANTS SUPPORT SPERM QUALITY

Antioxidants have a significant impact on sperm quality, largely due to their ability to reduce oxidative stress. Oxidation is a normal process that occurs in the body when oxygen combines with other molecules to produce energy. As sperm are produced, a healthy amount of oxidation takes place. Oxidation can also produce harmful by-products called free radicals, which can damage cells. Examples of this in everyday life include things like rust forming on a car. Thankfully, the body has a way of fighting this process (so no worries about rusty sperm!). Oxidative stress happens when there is an imbalance between free radicals and antioxidants in the body, and it impacts sperm anatomy as well as the amount of damage to sperm DNA. The good news is that antioxidants neutralize these harmful molecules and protect cells from damage. We address oxidative stress and its impact on sperm quality throughout this book. We look at both sides of the oxidative stress seesaw (see below) and discuss decreasing the factors that contribute to oxidation and increasing the body's access to antioxidants, which can be found in foods, supplements, and herbs.

THE OXIDATIVE STRESS SEESAW

To understand oxidative stress, think of it like a seesaw. On one side are things that contribute to oxidation, including normal cellular reactions, alcohol, stress, environmental exposures, aging, and more. On the other side are antioxidants. Oxidative stress occurs when antioxidants can't keep up with the stressors. It's all about balance. Our bodies have the amazing ability to keep oxidation in check when they have the right resources.

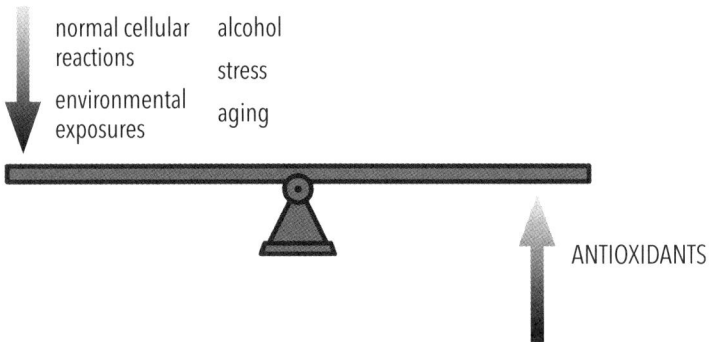

AGE AND SPERM HEALTH

We hear a lot about age being a factor for the ovulating partner, but what about the sperm-producing partner? Turns out, age matters for sperm, too. As a person gets older, sperm begin to experience problems with DNA fragmentation and single gene mutations, which can lead to difficulty getting pregnant, miscarriage, and long-term health issues for the baby. Research in this area is still emerging, and the exact age when these increased risks occur isn't clear, but most experts agree that sperm issues can be seen starting at age 40 and increase as a person ages.[1]

This age factor is yet another reason why supporting the fertility of both partners is crucial for getting pregnant, staying pregnant, and the future health of your baby.

CHAPTER 4

TIMING
IS EVERYTHING

· ·

Identifying and Maximizing
Your Fertile Window

Timing is everything, as the saying goes, and this
couldn't be more true when it comes to conception.
You can have a positive mindset, all the right pieces
and parts, and a good plan, but if you don't time things
correctly, it's unlikely you'll become pregnant.

Identifying Your Fertile Window

Did you know you have about 6 days each month when you can get pregnant? This is because sperm can live in the fallopian tubes for as long as 5 days, while an egg can survive for 12–24 hours after ovulation. This 6-day period is referred to as your fertile window. The ovulating partner is at their most fertile the day before and the day they ovulate. However, because sperm can survive up to 5 days, having sex on the days leading up to ovulation can increase your chances of getting pregnant. Once the egg has passed (usually within a day of ovulation), you cannot get pregnant until after the next menstrual cycle has started.

One of the biggest mistakes I see couples make is waiting until they think they've ovulated to have sex. They miss out on the 5 days prior to ovulation where sperm could hang out, waiting for the egg. Or, because an egg only lives for 12–24 hours, they miss the window entirely. For example, if you ovulated at 6:00 a.m. and that particular egg only lives 12 hours, if you have sex that evening, it will be too late.

Tracking Changes in Hormone Levels

So how do you know when you are in your fertile window? Let's start by reviewing what you learned in Chapter 2 about the menstrual cycle and ovulation. There are two main hormones involved in predicting ovulation during the first half of the cycle: estrogen and luteinizing hormone (LH). During each cycle, ovaries recruit many follicles to start maturing, one of which will reach full maturity and ovulate a mature egg.

Rising estrogen levels. As the dominant follicle containing the maturing egg starts growing, it produces estrogen. Rising estrogen levels during the first half of the cycle are the first sign that ovulation is coming, typically within the next 5 days.

Once estrogen reaches a high enough level, a signal is sent to the brain that the egg is mature and ready for ovulation. The brain then sends an LH surge to the ovary to trigger the follicle to rupture and release the egg. Ovulation typically occurs 12–36 hours after an LH surge. After ovulation, the follicle turns into a corpus luteum and produces progesterone.

The strategies in this chapter will help you identify the rise in estrogen (the start of your fertile window) and the LH surge (suggesting that ovulation is about to happen), and confirm that ovulation occurred (end of fertile window).

COMMON CONCEPTION MYTHS . . . BUSTED

MYTH: It's possible to get pregnant at any time of the month.
FACT: You can only get pregnant in your fertile window, which is typically 5–6 days of the month.

MYTH: You can conceive only on 2 days each cycle.
FACT: The egg will only survive for 12–24 hours after ovulation, but sperm can live for up to 5 days, resulting in a 5-day window each month.

MYTH: Tracking the ovulating partner's morning temperature can help you time intercourse and get pregnant quickly.
FACT: Body temperature rises *after* ovulation, indicating it is too late for conception this month. (But tracking your temp is still helpful! More on that later in this chapter.)

MYTH: The best way to time intercourse is to wait for confirmation of ovulation.
FACT: Because the egg only lives for 12–24 hours after ovulation, waiting may cause you to miss the egg.

MYTH: Having sex on cycle day 14 will increase your chances of getting pregnant.
FACT: A person could ovulate as early as cycle day 8, as late as day 20, or later! Most people don't actually ovulate on day 14.

MYTH: Frequent intercourse decreases sperm. It's best to "save it up" for ovulation.
FACT: Studies show that if sperm quality is normal, abstinence does not increase the chance of pregnancy and, in fact, could decrease sperm quality.

Observing Cervical Fluid

Cervical fluid (also called cervical mucus) is produced by the cervix during certain days of the cycle and is essential for conception as it creates the ideal environment for sperm. Sperm depend on cervical fluid for survival, movement, and to prepare for fertilization. Without this fluid, the sperm simply cannot reach or fertilize the egg.

Cervical fluid occurs naturally and regularly and is one of the first indicators that you are in your fertile window. It can be a powerful tool for knowing when to time intercourse. You are only fertile on the days you observe cervical fluid, so knowing what to look for is key.

Here's how to recognize fertile days throughout the month:

Dry days. The start of a cycle begins with a period. After menstruation ends, you will typically have a few days without any cervical fluid, also referred to as dry days. These are nonfertile days.

Possible but not ideal days. As estrogen rises and the ovary prepares for ovulation, you will notice the start of cervical mucus. This is often sticky or pasty. This is technically the start of your fertile window, although this consistency of cervical mucus is not the most conducive to sperm survival (but it is possible!). This is referred to as nonpeak cervical fluid.

Getting closer. As estrogen continues to rise, cervical fluid takes on a wetter consistency. It becomes creamy, similar to hand lotion. Still referred to as nonpeak cervical fluid, this is within your fertile window, with a good chance for sperm to survive long enough to fertilize the egg over the next few days.

Peak fertile days. The final and most fertile cervical mucus is even more wet, stretchy, clear, and slippery, similar to the look and feel of raw egg whites. This is considered peak cervical fluid, meaning you are close to ovulation and in your peak fertility days.

Back to dry days. After ovulation, cervical fluid shifts back to dry or absent as it forms a thick mucous plug inside your cervical canal, acting as a barrier to block sperm from entering the uterus. These are nonfertile days and will last until the start of your next cycle.

Not all people observe cervical fluid changes exactly as described. The important thing to remember is that if you see any cervical mucus, you are in your fertile window, and egg white consistency marks your peak fertile window.

HOW TO CHECK YOUR CERVICAL FLUID

So how do you check your cervical fluid? The easiest way is for the ovulating partner to check every time they go to the bathroom: Get into the habit of wiping before urinating and notice what is on the toilet paper. If there is any fluid on the paper, you are in your fertile window. Dry paper indicates nonfertile days.

Many people are surprised by how checking cervical fluid can become second nature, and the information that it provides for timing intercourse is invaluable.

DETERMINING FERTILE DAYS BASED ON CERVICAL FLUID

	NONFERTILE		FERTILE (5-6 DAYS)		NONFERTILE
PHASE	Menstruation	No cervical fluid	Nonpeak cervical fluid	Peak cervical fluid	No cervical fluid
SIGN	Menstrual flow	Absent or dry	Sticky, creamy, or lotion quality	Clear, stretchy, slippery, or egg white quality	Absent or dry

PRODUCTS AND PRACTICES THAT
NEGATIVELY AFFECT CERVICAL FLUID

Douching. Vaginal douching can wash away the cervical mucus you need to get pregnant. Douching can also alter the microbiome of the vagina, leading to an increased risk of vaginal infection.

Lubricants. Sexual lubricants can change the pH of the vagina, harm sperm, and disrupt cervical fluid. Look for lubricants that specifically say they are "fertility friendly." Be aware they can make it harder to notice your own cervical fluid.

Dehydration. It sounds simple, but staying hydrated is important for overall health and bodily fluids, including cervical fluid. Peak cervical fluid is 90 percent water.

Antihistamines or allergy medications. Cold and allergy medications can decrease cervical fluid just like they dry up nasal mucus. Usually, drugs like these are taken for a limited period of time and are not a problem, but if you are taking a long-term dosage or notice a change in your cervical fluid, it may be worth finding alternatives. Check out my recipe for Simple Overnight Nettle Infusion (page 91), which has a side benefit of helping decrease allergies when taken regularly over several months.

Oral contraceptives. If you were recently on birth control pills, it can take a few months for cervical fluid to return.

Age. It's normal to notice a decrease in cervical fluid as you age, including a decrease in the number of peak fertile days.

Nutritional deficiencies. A healthy diet full of antioxidants and vitamins can help maintain a healthy cervix and cervical fluid.

Over-the-Counter Ovulation Detection

Ovulation predictor kits (OPKs), sometimes referred to as LH or ovulation test strips, are a popular method for determining when to time intercourse. OPKs work by measuring levels of LH in your urine. Remember, a rise in LH signals the ovary to release an egg. When levels reach a certain threshold, there is a positive indication on the test strip and ovulation typically occurs within the next 12–36 hours. OPKs can provide valuable information, but there are several limitations to only using this method to predict your fertile window.

OPK LIMITATIONS

You will miss the full fertile window. OPKs typically identify the 2 days when the ovulating partner is most fertile. Now that you understand what is happening with cervical mucus as estrogen rises, you know that you have a 5- to 6-day window where you can get pregnant. Using an OPK alone means you will miss out on the days before the LH spike when your fertile window begins.

You could be too late. For at least 30 percent of people,[1] ovulation occurs on the same day as their LH surge. This means if you were to have sex only on the day you got the positive ovulation test, you may have missed ovulation completely.

Doesn't confirm ovulation really happened. A surge in LH levels indicates that ovulation should take place, but in some cases, ovulation doesn't happen in the expected time frame or at all.

Not reliable for people with polycystic ovary syndrome (PCOS). Because LH can be elevated at other times of the month with PCOS, this produces false positives leading to confusion over when to have intercourse.

Cost. Test strips can be expensive, especially if you have a long or irregular cycle and need to test for multiple days to find the peak.

So how do OPKs fit into a holistic fertility plan? Used in combination with tracking cervical fluid, OPKs can provide helpful information. The LH surge should occur around the same time that you notice peak cervical fluid (wet, slippery, or egg white). When you first start monitoring, you may have a hard time distinguishing between fertile mucus and peak fertile mucus, and seeing the LH surge may help to differentiate. As you get more familiar with the tracking process, you will notice your fertile window starts several days before your LH surge. OPKs are simply another tool we can use to increase your chances of getting pregnant; they can provide additional information to help you identify your peak fertile days but should not be relied on exclusively.

TIPS FOR USING OPKs

- Start testing the day after a period ends.

- Use LH strips late morning through early evening (between 12 p.m. and 6 p.m. is best) for optimal timing.

- Test twice a day, since the surge can rise and fall quickly.

- Avoid overhydration, which can dilute hormones.

- Once you get a positive LH surge, you can stop testing.

The Truth About Temperature

The most common misconception about tracking basal body temperature (BBT) is that it can help *predict* when someone is going to ovulate in order to better time intercourse. In reality, BBT is an extremely helpful way to *confirm* ovulation *after* it has occurred. This is a useful piece of the fertility puzzle, but it isn't useful for timing intercourse for conception in a current cycle.

Tracking BBT is a bit like a postgame analysis. It lets us know that the main event (ovulation) really did occur, and gives us valuable information about the postovulatory, or luteal, phase of the cycle. This information allows us to gather more details important to your fertility.

When you measure BBT each morning, you will notice a clear difference between temperatures before and after ovulation. This is because after ovulation progesterone levels rise, which increases body temperature enough to shift BBT, and remains high for the rest of the cycle. If you are not pregnant, temperatures will drop back down to preovulatory levels 12–16 days after the rise, and a period will start. If you are pregnant, BBT will remain elevated throughout the entire pregnancy due to elevated progesterone levels.

Because BBT rises *after* ovulation has taken place, and your fertile window is the 6 days leading up to and including ovulation, once temperature rises it's usually too late to conceive.

How to Track Temperature

Take the ovulating partner's temperature orally at the same time each morning upon waking and before getting out of bed or doing anything else. To confirm ovulation, you need three consecutive temperatures that are 0.04–1.0°F higher than the previous six preovulatory temperatures (assuming temperatures are not abnormally high due to illness or other factors). A BBT thermometer is recommended, as it can track temperature in increments of hundredths of a degree. This thermometer is faster and more exact than a regular thermometer, and can be purchased at most drugstores and online.

If the idea of methodically taking your temperature every morning, before getting out of bed, sounds like a pain, there are some great alternatives in the form of wearable products (rings to wear on a finger, under-the-arm temperature monitors, etc.) that will take average temperature over time. This is technically not a BBT, but it is still relevant for confirming ovulation and monitoring postovulatory phase. The same principle applies—look for a clear shift from consistent lower temperatures to consistent higher temperatures to confirm that ovulation has occurred.

BRINGING IT ALL TOGETHER: CHARTING YOUR CYCLES

The trifecta for optimal "getting pregnant" conditions is cervical fluid, LH surge, and BBT.

From this chart we can see the following.

- Cervical fluid appeared on day 14, marking the start of the fertile window.

- Cervical fluid shifted from creamy to egg white on days 17 and 18, indicating peak fertile days.

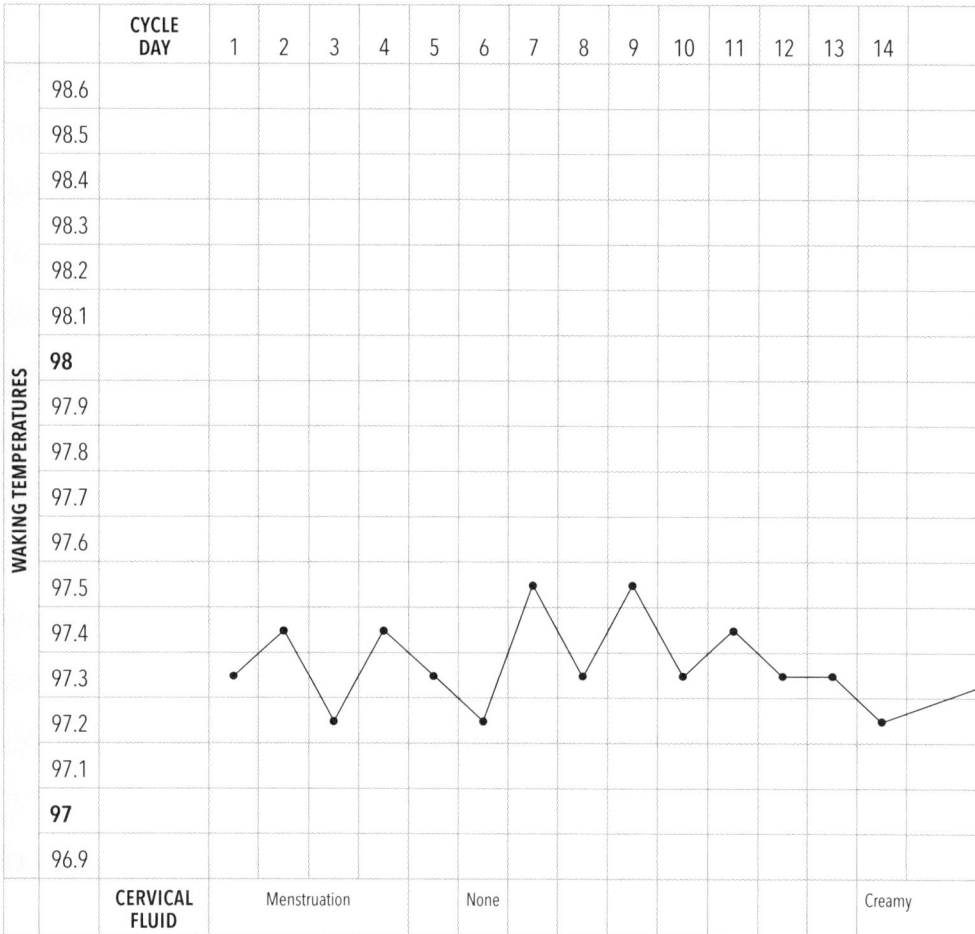

		CYCLE DAY	1	2	3	4	5	6	7	8	9	10	11	12	13	14	
WAKING TEMPERATURES	98.6																
	98.5																
	98.4																
	98.3																
	98.2																
	98.1																
	98																
	97.9																
	97.8																
	97.7																
	97.6																
	97.5								•		•						
	97.4			•		•							•				
	97.3		•				•			•				•	•		
	97.2				•			•								•	
	97.1																
	97																
	96.9																
	CERVICAL FLUID		Menstruation				None								Creamy		

- OPK showed "positive" on day 18, indicating ovulation should occur in the next 12–24 hours.
- Cervical fluid was absent on day 19, indicating the end of the fertile window.
- BBT was elevated on day 19, confirming ovulation occurred the day before (cycle day 18).

- Temperatures stayed elevated for 14 days before the start of the next menstrual cycle, indicating a luteal phase long enough for implantation to occur, but no pregnancy this month.
- Total cycle length was 32 days.

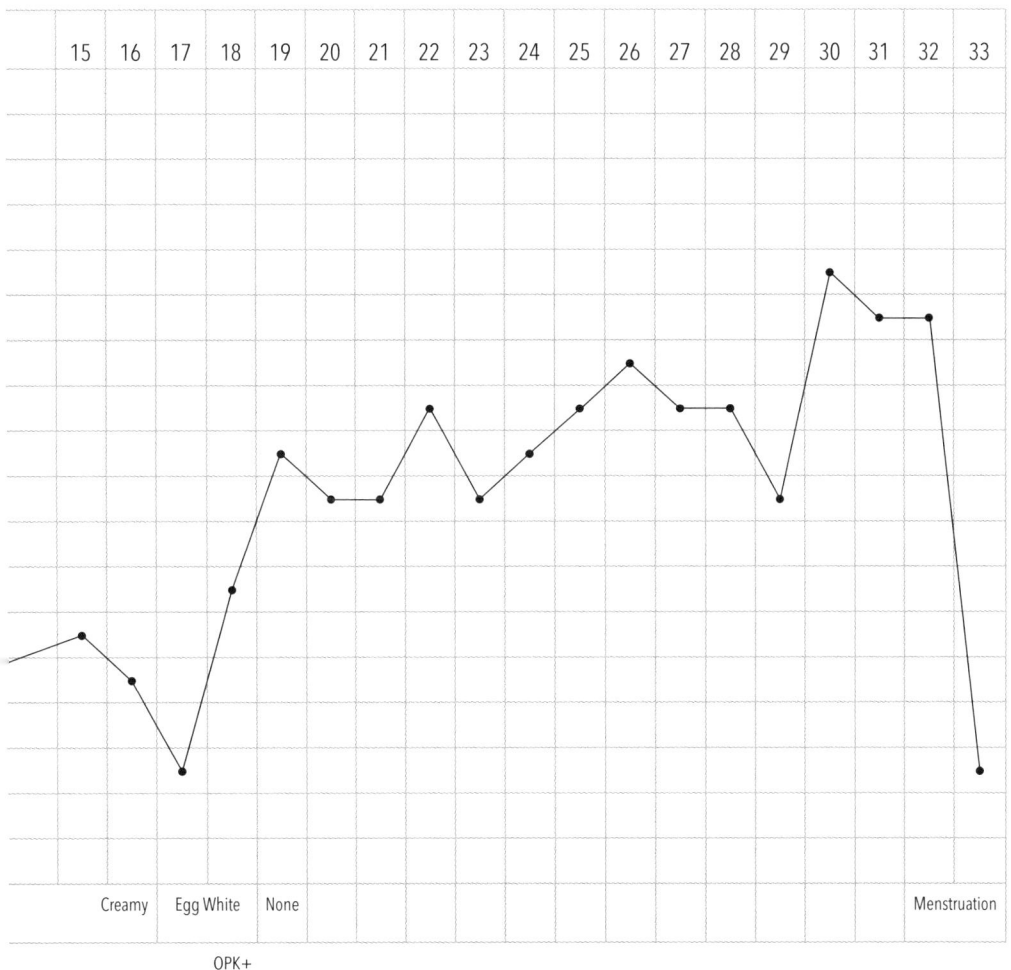

| 15 | 16 | 17 | 18 | 19 | 20 | 21 | 22 | 23 | 24 | 25 | 26 | 27 | 28 | 29 | 30 | 31 | 32 | 33 |

Creamy   Egg White   None   Menstruation

OPK+

OTHER INFORMATION TEMPERATURE TRACKING PROVIDES

In addition to confirming ovulation, tracking temperatures in the second half of a cycle can provide valuable information. Once temperature rises, the length of time until the next period will remain fairly consistent from cycle to cycle, and will generally last between 12 and 16 days. Most people's luteal phase doesn't vary more than 1–2 days. Knowing how long your luteal phase typically lasts provides the following information:

Predicting when to expect the next period. If you know your luteal phase is consistently 12 days, then even with irregular cycles, you can predict when a period is due.

Detecting a pregnancy. Monitoring luteal phase temperatures will help you know when to test for pregnancy. It's a good sign you might be pregnant if you've had 18 days of elevated temperatures.

Luteal phase too short for implantation. If temperature is not elevated for 10 days before your period, it could mean that your luteal phase isn't long enough for an embryo to implant (more on short luteal phase in Chapter 11).

OTHER FACTORS THAT CAN INCREASE BBT

When you start recording BBT or average temperatures from a wearable device, be aware of events other than ovulation that can elevate temperature. While this may seem confusing at first, look at the general trend of temperatures. Make a note of things happening in your life that may have triggered the fluctuation. Some of these might include:

- Illness

- Alcohol

- Poor sleep quality

- Inconsistent monitoring of temperature (time of day and devices)

- Stress

- Travel, time changes, jet lag

- Sleeping with a heating pad or electric blanket

How Often Should You Have Sex?

Now that you are clear on when to time intercourse, the next question is how often. There are loads of opinions, rumors, and old wives' tales that can create confusion, stress, or worry, which totally takes the fun out of it! Thankfully, we have research to help make informed decisions. Here's the truth about how often to have intercourse.

The biggest debate is whether you should have intercourse every day or every other day in your fertile window. Don't drive yourself crazy trying to figure out the perfect timing. I'll tell you what I tell my clients: *Take the pressure off yourselves!* And here's why. Research shows daily intercourse during the fertile window resulted in a 37 percent pregnancy rate, while every-other-day intercourse had a 33 percent pregnancy rate. That is a very small difference. Even having sex only once during the fertile window resulted in a 15 percent pregnancy rate,[2] so relax and enjoy being together every day, every other day, or even just once during the fertile window.

Another popular myth is that frequent intercourse decreases sperm. A study of almost 10,000 people with normal sperm found that daily ejaculation did not hinder sperm parameters.[3] However, abstinence of 10 days or more did begin to deteriorate sperm quality.[4] Intercourse every other day in the fertile window is just as effective as every day, and the optimal frequency of intercourse is whatever works for you and your partner within that context. Don't worry about "overuse" and don't "save it up" for too long.

KEY POINTS FOR FERTILITY AWARENESS AND TIMING INTERCOURSE

You are fertile for about 6 days each month: 5 days before ovulation and the day of ovulation. The key to identifying your fertile window is monitoring cervical fluid.

- Dry = not fertile
- Presence of cervical fluid = fertile
- Wet or egg white = peak fertile window

Have intercourse every day or every other day from the start of cervical fluid until it ends (confirmed by elevated temperature).

A rise in temperature of 0.04–1.0°F above baseline confirms ovulation occurred the previous day.

The luteal phase (the days the ovulating partner's temperature is elevated) will remain relatively consistent and can help you predict when a next period is expected, if you could be pregnant, or if the luteal phase is too short for implantation.

CHAPTER 5

FERTILITY TESTING

···

Understanding What to Test and Why

There's nothing more frustrating than trying to conceive for months without knowing if there's something hindering your chances of pregnancy. Understanding your basic fertility status can ease your worries and help you take proactive steps toward realizing your family goals. So why wait? Early fertility testing gives you the knowledge to make informed decisions about your reproductive health and family planning journey. While deeper evaluations by a reproductive endocrinologist or reproductive urologist might require a referral, you shouldn't have to wait for the basic blood work or sperm testing suggested in this chapter. Your primary care doctor or gynecologist can order these tests for you.

Testing for Eggs, Ovulation, and Cycle Hormones

Remember the hormonal dance that occurs every month to build up the uterine lining, develop a follicle, release an egg, and menstruate? Measuring these precise hormone levels at specific times in the cycle will give us valuable insights into your fertility.

Fertility blood work for the ovulating partner can be broken down into three categories: blood work that is drawn early in your menstrual cycle (cycle day 3), blood work that is drawn after ovulation (7–10 days after ovulation), and blood work that can be done at any time. Timing is key because testing on the wrong day will give inaccurate and irrelevant results.

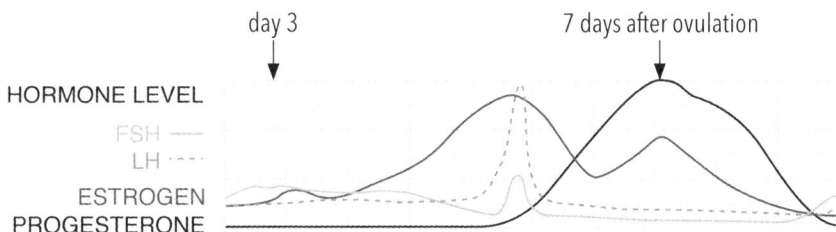

Day 3 Blood Work

Day 3 blood work needs to be drawn early in your cycle, ideally on cycle day 3, but definitely sometime during days 2 through 4. Cycle day 1 is the first day of your period. You count day 1 as the first day you experience full flow, not just spotting, before 5 p.m. Full flow means enough that you need a menstrual product. For example, if you have spotting on Monday, but full flow requiring a tampon on Tuesday, then Tuesday is day 1 and Thursday will be day 3. Days 2–4 are okay for testing as long as you're still experiencing flow. If you have a short period (lasting fewer than 3 days), then test on day 2.

FOLLICLE-STIMULATING HORMONE (FSH)

FSH is a hormone sent by the brain to the ovaries, signaling them to start growing follicles, each containing an egg. Imagine it's the kick-off for a team of tiny eggs in your ovaries! As follicles grow, they produce the hormone estradiol. The brain and ovaries talk to each other. If everything is going well and the ovaries are responding, the follicles grow and make more estradiol. But if the ovaries aren't doing their job properly and the follicles aren't making enough estradiol, the brain sends more FSH to give them a nudge.

When FSH levels are high, it tells us that the ovaries might need some extra encouragement. In other words, this test helps answer the question "Are the ovaries responding to the brain or does the brain need to shout a bit louder for a response?" Elevated levels are associated with diminished ovarian function, a reduced egg count, premature ovarian failure, and menopause.

Ranges: 9 mIU/L is considered optimal, and 15–18 mIU/L is unlikely to respond to IVF but still possible to ovulate and conceive naturally. Elevated estrogen can suppress FSH. If your estradiol levels are above 50 pg/mL then FSH may not be an accurate indicator of ovarian function.

ESTRADIOL

Estradiol (sometimes shown on medical reports as "E2") is the hormone released by the granulosa cells of the developing follicles. It increases gradually from the beginning of the menstrual cycle until the point of ovulation. The level of estradiol reflects how big and mature the egg-containing follicles are. This hormone plays an important role in egg maturation, production of cervical fluid, and thickening the uterus lining for an embryo to attach.

Typically, estradiol levels are low on cycle day 3, showing that follicles are just beginning to develop. However, higher levels could mean there are fewer eggs, causing the body to speed up its response to FSH to make up for the shortfall, or could suggest ovarian cysts. As ovarian aging continues and egg reserves decrease, the brain has to work harder to get the ovaries to respond (by increasing FSH); eventually, the ovaries stop altogether and estradiol levels drop.

Day 3 estradiol helps answer the question "Are the follicles starting to develop as expected?" Low estradiol could indicate premature ovarian insufficiency, hypothalamic amenorrhea, or menopause.

Ranges: Between 30 and 50 pg/mL is considered optimal. Keep in mind that estradiol and FSH levels work in opposition: When estrogen levels increase, FSH levels decrease. Therefore, an estradiol level above 50 pg/mL can actually suppress FSH, potentially leading to an inaccurate assessment.

LUTEINIZING HORMONE (LH)

LH is produced by the pituitary gland and plays a crucial role in triggering ovulation. At the beginning of the menstrual cycle, LH levels are relatively low. It's only when estrogen levels rise enough to signal an egg is ready for release that LH starts to spike.

This surge in LH is essential for the start of ovulation and is what home ovulation predictor kits detect. FSH and LH communicate with each other, so it's important to note their relationship. If LH is significantly higher than FSH, it could be a sign of polycystic ovary syndrome (PCOS). On the other hand, low LH levels may indicate hypothalamic amenorrhea, often linked to excessive exercise or insufficient caloric intake.

Ranges: Day 3 LH should be in a 1:1 ratio with FSH and be less than 7 mIU/mL. If LH is twice as high as FSH, it might suggest PCOS. Elevated LH levels, typically greater than 15 mIU/mL, could indicate premature ovarian insufficiency, menopause, or, in cases of very short menstrual cycles, the beginning of the LH surge and early ovulation.

After Ovulation Blood Work

Progesterone levels are tested 7–10 days after ovulation. Testing before ovulation or too soon after doesn't provide any meaningful information. How do you determine when to test? Once you confirm ovulation, either by using an OPK, recording a rise in basal body temperature, or noticing changes in cervical fluid, then count ahead 7–10 days to schedule your progesterone test. For example, if you know ovulation occurred on cycle day 16, then test progesterone 7–10 days later, on cycle day 23, 24, 25, or 26.

Many providers will tell you to test progesterone on day 21 of a cycle, but this is only accurate if ovulation occurred around day 14 (14 + 7 = 21). If ovulation was earlier or later than day 14, your results will be skewed.

PROGESTERONE

The main function of progesterone (sometimes shown on reports as "P4") is to help a pregnancy by supporting the uterine lining until the placenta can take over. Before ovulation, progesterone levels are barely detectable. After ovulation, the follicle turns into a corpus luteum and produces large amounts of progesterone for about 14 days, or longer if pregnant.

Testing progesterone at the correct time (7–10 days after ovulation) helps answer the question "Did ovulation occur and is progesterone high enough to maintain a pregnancy?"

Ranges: 10 ng/mL or greater is a good progesterone level; some providers prefer to see >15 ng/mL. Any level above 4 ng/mL is a reasonable assurance that ovulation occurred. Progesterone fluctuates widely over the course of 90 minutes, so a low-normal reading may simply mean the blood was drawn at a low point and should be retested.

Any Day Blood Work

These tests can be performed any day of the cycle and are typically done at the same time as the day 3 blood work for convenience.

ANTI-MÜLLERIAN HORMONE (AMH)

Anti-Müllerian hormone (AMH) is made in the cells of developing follicles. Therefore, more follicles mean higher AMH levels, and more eggs. AMH is a good indication of how many eggs are in development but isn't useful in predicting your overall chances of becoming pregnant, nor does it give any indication of egg quality.

If you are going through an IVF cycle, AMH can be associated with the number of eggs that will be available for retrieval.

Testing your AMH can help answer the question "How many eggs do I have right now?"

Ranges: Normal AMH ranges depend on age, but in general, an optimal AMH is between 2 and 4 ng/mL. Higher AMH could indicate PCOS and warrants further workup.

PROLACTIN

The prolactin hormone, which is normally associated with things happening after pregnancy (i.e., regulating lactation), can increase with stress, certain medications, pituitary tumors, PCOS, and hypothyroidism. High prolactin levels can suppress FSH and LH, disrupting ovulation and the entire hormonal process.

Testing prolactin helps answer the question "Is this hormone too high for me to get pregnant?"

Ranges: Less than 20 ng/mL

THYROID-STIMULATING HORMONE (TSH)

TSH is produced by the pituitary gland and tells the thyroid how much thyroid hormone it needs to make. When thyroid hormone levels drop, the pituitary gland increases TSH production to prompt the thyroid to work harder. On the flip side, if thyroid hormone levels rise, TSH production decreases. By measuring TSH levels in your blood, you can find out if your thyroid is making the right levels. Thyroid imbalances can have a major impact on fertility.

Testing TSH helps answer the question "Is my thyroid in optimal range for fertility?"

Ranges: 0.45–2.5 mIU/L. The optimal range for fertility should be more narrowly managed than it is for general health: A full thyroid panel with antibodies can be helpful, especially if TSH is out of optimal range or borderline.

DHEA-SULFATE (DHEA-S)

Dehydroepiandrosterone (DHEA), made by the adrenal glands, acts as a building block for different hormones, including testosterone and estrogen. As a person ages or experiences a decline in ovarian reserve, DHEA-S levels typically decrease, while they tend to rise in cases of PCOS. If the ovulating partner doesn't have enough of this hormone, it leads to lower testosterone and estrogen levels, which affect the quality of eggs.

Testing DHEA-S helps answer the question "Do I have enough of this hormone to support egg quality?"

Ranges: The normal ranges vary based on age, but generally 120–279 mcg/dL is considered optimal. It is helpful to test DHEA-S and testosterone together.

TESTOSTERONE (TOTAL AND FREE) FOR OVULATING PARTNER

Testosterone is an important hormone for helping follicles grow and ensuring good egg quality. As we age, testosterone naturally declines, which can affect egg quality. Elevated levels of testosterone are often associated with PCOS.

Most testosterone floats around in the bloodstream bound to other proteins and is "locked up" and can't really have an effect on the body. Free testosterone, on the other hand, is unbound and active. Testing both total and free testosterone provides a more complete picture.

Testing total and free testosterone helps answer the question "Do I have enough of this hormone to support egg quality, but not too much?"

Ranges: Total testosterone: 32–60 ng/dL; free testosterone: 0.3–1.9 ng/dL

25-HYDROXYVITAMIN D (25[OH]D)

Vitamin D is important both for getting and for staying pregnant, as well as your overall health. Testing vitamin D levels helps answer the question "Are my levels sufficient for optimal fertility and healthy pregnancy?"

Ranges: 30–50 ng/mL. Although there's still debate about the optimal levels of vitamin D, most labs in the United States use 30 ng/mL as the cutoff for normal. However, studies suggest that levels between 30 and 50 ng/mL may be more beneficial for fertility.

A word of caution when looking at your own test results: Don't fixate on one suboptimal number. Keep in mind that hormones fluctuate, even varying throughout the day, so if some tests come back wonky, it's worth repeating them again the following month.

It's also key to realize that reference ranges are just that—a reference—and your fertility is influenced by numerous factors. Making sweeping assumptions based on a single test outcome isn't accurate or helpful. It's so important to look at the bigger picture—consider the full range of lab work and your overall health, and, please, make sure you talk with a professional to help you interpret the results.

In my own practice, I've witnessed people positively influence their blood test numbers simply by incorporating changes to their diet and lifestyle by adding things like herbs and supplements, making nutritional adjustments, and reducing exposure to certain chemicals. Small changes made consistently can have a positive impact on fertility health.

Testing for Sperm and Testosterone

Have you been told your sperm parameters are normal but not optimal? This can impact your overall fertility and the time it takes to achieve a pregnancy.

Before we dive into what is considered normal, low, and optimal, let's first take a step back and discuss how sperm is analyzed. A semen analysis is the most common test to evaluate sperm parameters and is considered the gold-standard assessment for the workup of sperm-related infertility. Newer tests that look at DNA fragmentation can be useful for deeper analysis of the sperm.

Semen Analysis

The parameters reported in a semen analysis can be grouped into three main categories: how much, how well they swim, and how they look.

HOW MUCH?

This refers to how much semen, in volume, and how many sperm. Common parameters listed in a semen analysis report are:

- Semen volume: the total amount of ejaculate in milliliters

- Sperm count: the total number of sperm in the semen sample

- Sperm concentration: measurement of how many million sperm in each milliliter of semen

HOW WELL DO THEY SWIM?

In order for fertilization to occur, sperm need to progress from the vagina, through the cervix and uterus, and into the fallopian tubes to penetrate and fertilize the egg. Even in assisted reproductive procedures such as IVF or IUI, the sperm still need to swim to meet and fertilize the egg. While this is a complex process, at its most basic level, the sperm needs to swim to its target. This is referred to as motility. Common parameters listed are:

- Progressive motility (PR): the percentage of sperm that are swimming in a predominantly straight line or in very large circles

- Nonprogressive motility (NP): the percentage of sperm that move but don't make forward progression, or swim in very tight circles

- Total motility (PR + NP): the percentage of sperm that are moving in the semen sample; includes progressive (PR) and nonprogressive (NP) motility

HOW DO THEY LOOK?

Normal sperm have an oval head with a long tail. This is referred to as morphology. Sperm can be misshaped based on the size of the head, having an extra head, and having no head or tail. These defects could affect the ability of the sperm to reach and penetrate an egg. Surprisingly, it is common for the majority of sperm per ejaculate to be abnormally formed. Common parameters listed are:

- Morphology: the percentage of sperm that have "normal" size and shape, and may also be called "normal forms"

- Vitality: the percentage of live, membrane-intact sperm

A problem in any one of these parameters will make it more difficult to conceive.

SEMEN ANALYSIS GLOSSARY OF TERMS

Oligospermia: low sperm count, fewer than 15 million sperm per milliliter

Azoospermia: a complete absence of any sperm

Normospermia: normal sperm count

Asthenospermia: reduced sperm motility (movement), also known as asthenozoospermia; less than 40 percent of sperm with motility or less than 32 percent with progressive motility

Teratospermia: poor morphology (shape), also known as teratozoospermia; less than 4 percent of sperm have a normal shape

Aspermia: complete lack of semen during ejaculation—no fluid is released

Semen Parameters

Most labs report semen parameters using values established by the World Health Organization (WHO), which is based on data collected and published in 2010.[1] The WHO study reviewed semen samples from more than 4,500 people from 14 countries and included people whose partners became pregnant within 12 months of stopping the use of contraception.

PARAMETERS (UNITS)	WHO NORMAL RANGE
Semen volume (mL)	1.5–6.8 mL
Sperm count (per ejaculate) Total number of sperm in the semen sample	39–802 million
Sperm concentration (per mL) Measurement of how many million sperm in each milliliter of semen	15–213 million
Total motility (PR + NP) The percentage of sperm that are moving in the semen sample; includes progressive (PR) and nonprogressive (NP) motility	40–78%
Progressive motility (PR) The percentage of sperm that are swimming in a mostly straight line or in very large circles	32–72%
Nonprogressive motility (NP) The percentage of sperm that move but don't make forward progression, or swim in very tight circles	1–18%
Vitality The percentage of sperm that is alive	58–91%
Morphology (normal forms) The percentage of sperm that have "normal" size and shape	4–44%

From: WHO Normal Values Chart (World Health Organization, 2010)

Semen Analysis: Normal versus Optimal

As you can see from the chart above, there is a wide range of what is considered normal. Because the normal range represents *all people whose partner became pregnant within 12 months of stopping the use of contraception*, it's helpful to expand the data into percentiles. Each percentile answers the question "What percentage of the fertile group had this particular sperm parameter?" Anything between the 5th to the 95th percentile is considered normal, but is it optimal?

Distribution of values for semen parameters from people whose partners become pregnant within 12 months:[2]

PARAMETER	5TH PERCENTILE	25TH PERCENTILE	50TH PERCENTILE	75TH PERCENTILE	95TH PERCENTILE
Sperm count (per ejaculate)	39 million	142 million	255 million	422 million	802 million
Sperm concentration (per mL)	15 million/mL	41 million/mL	73 million/mL	116 million/mL	213 million/mL
Total motility (PR + NP)	40%	53%	61%	69%	78%
Progressive motility (PR)	32%	47%	55%	62%	72%
Morphology (normal forms)	4%	9%	15%	24.5%	44%

THE LOWER END OF NORMAL

Let's take a closer look at the lower end of the normal range, which is represented by the 5th percentile. WHO found that 5 percent of the people who conceived within a year of stopping contraception had sperm concentrations that were 15 million/mL. That means that while it was possible to become pregnant with a sperm concentration of 15 million/mL, *only 5 percent* of the people in this fertile group were in that range.

Moving up the percentile chart you can see that 50 percent of the people who achieved pregnancy in this group had sperm concentrations that were 73 million/mL. Ninety-five percent of people who achieved pregnancy had sperm concentrations of 213 million/mL. In other words, *most people* who became pregnant had sperm parameters in the 50th percentile or higher.

Many experts advocate that optimal sperm parameters are values in the 50th percentile or higher, and studies show a faster time to pregnancy in this higher percentile range.[3,4] Of course, this data does not take into account egg quality, but it is a helpful guide when looking at sperm parameters and their impact on fertility.

Knowing where your sperm parameters fall on the percentile chart can help you understand if your parameters are normal or optimal, an important factor in how long it may take to become pregnant.

SPERM HEALTH AROUND THE WORLD:
ARE WE FACING A GLOBAL DECLINE?

Sperm health first made headlines when a meta-analysis (a study of past studies) reported a significant decline in sperm parameters. This study showed that sperm concentration declined 52.4 percent (–1.4 percent per year) between 1973 and 2011.[5] Sperm motility, a measure highly relevant to fertilization success, declined by approximately 10 percent between 2002 and 2017.[6,7]

In 1940, the average sperm concentration was 113 million sperm per milliliter of semen (million/mL). In 1990, the average had fallen to 66 million/mL.[8]

A large number of people have sperm concentrations below 40 million/mL, which is worrying because concentrations below this threshold are linked to a reduced likelihood of conception.[9]

Researchers are sounding the alarm: The disturbing decrease in sperm quality and fertility is now escalating into a broader fertility crisis.[10] The reason for this global decline in sperm parameters is still being studied, but lifestyle factors such as illicit drug use, smoking, poor nutrition, stress, and genetic factors all play a role. Exposure to everyday chemicals appears to have a significant impact (and is something we can control—more on that in Chapter 10). Plastics, pesticides, and artificial fragrances have all been shown to have a serious impact on sperm quality.[11]

Sperm DNA Fragmentation

While a semen analysis provides information regarding sperm count, mobility, and morphology, it will not provide insights regarding the quality of the DNA within sperm. Sperm DNA fragmentation (SDF) has emerged as a new testing tool to look inside the sperm to assess the quality of its DNA. An SDF test specifically looks at how many physical breaks are present in the DNA strands.

If the sperm's DNA is damaged, it reduces the chance of pregnancy and a healthy baby. Research shows that high levels of DNA fragmentation in sperm is associated with infertility, failure of IVF treatment, and early miscarriage. While experts disagree on specific cutoff values, generally speaking, an SDF over 30 percent is considered high and could have a negative impact on fertility.

A DNA fragmentation test can detect male fertility issues that may be missed during a traditional semen analysis. Consider SDF testing if you have a diagnosis of unexplained infertility, if you have had two or more miscarriages, or if the sperm-producing partner is over 40 years old.

The more information you have about sperm quality the better. We know that environmental factors such as heat exposure, environmental toxins, radiation, smoking, drug abuse, and poor diet lead to more DNA fragmentation.[12] The good news is the strategies in this book will help you minimize these environmental factors and help support your body to repair damage.

Improving sperm quality is even more important when egg quality is a concern. Eggs have the unique ability to repair DNA damage after fertilization, overcoming some of the negative effects of damaged sperm.[13] Pretty amazing that a healthy egg could compensate for some level of sperm DNA damage, resulting in a healthy embryo!

Does Sperm Quality Even Matter for IVF?

A common belief is that sperm quality doesn't matter when using assisted reproductive procedures such as IVF or IVF with intracytoplasmic sperm injection (ICSI). In theory, this belief makes sense, considering the sperm are placed in a petri dish close to the egg or injected directly into the egg. While the total number of sperm and how well they swim are less critical, research shows that sperm quality and health still contribute to a healthy embryo and successful pregnancy. If you are planning on using IVF or IVF with ICSI, use the strategies in this book to help improve your odds.

In the big picture, there is more to sperm quality than meets the eye (or is analyzed in a semen analysis), and it's important to understand that supporting the sperm's overall health will increase your fertility success rate no matter how you are going about it.

Other Tests for Sperm-Producing Partners

TESTOSTERONE

As discussed in Chapter 3, testosterone is the primary hormone involved in sperm production. Maintaining normal concentrations of testosterone promotes sperm production, whereas low levels of testosterone can lead to infertility. A simple blood test to look at testosterone levels provides important information regarding how to support optimal sperm quality. Testing for testosterone levels should be done between 7 and 10 a.m., as this is when levels are at their highest.

Ranges: Total testosterone reference ranges are typically between 300 and 1,000 ng/dL. Optimal levels are >450 ng/dL.

Free testosterone reference range is between 66 and 272 pg/mL. Optimal range is >98 pg/mL.

JACK'S STORY
Deciding to Test Sperm

Here's a story about Jack and his partner, who had been trying to conceive for 3 years. Having just finished their first IVF cycle, they were disappointed to learn that after having several eggs retrieved and fertilized, only one embryo made it to transfer day and ultimately did not result in a pregnancy. According to their lab tests, everything was normal. The diagnosis: unexplained infertility. Prescription: another round of IVF.

SUBOPTIMAL SPERM PARAMETERS

When I first met with the couple, they told me they wanted to take a few months to optimize their health and fertility before going through another round of IVF. After reviewing their lab results, one area stood out. Jack had been told his semen analysis was normal, but in reality, his sperm parameters were at the very low end of normal and were far from optimal. When I discussed this with Jack and his partner, they were surprised to learn there was a difference between normal and optimal semen parameters.

Jack's sperm concentration (the amount of sperm) was 128 m/mL, putting him in the optimal category. That's the good news! But his total motility (percentage of sperm swimming in any direction) was 40 percent, the very bottom of normal range. His progressive motility (percentage of sperm swimming in mostly a straight line) was 28 percent, slightly under the 5th percentile. And morphology (the percentage of sperm with a normal shape) was 4 percent, again in the 5th percentile.

GETTING JACK'S SWIMMERS BACK ON TRACK

So while Jack had an optimal amount of sperm, his sperm motility and morphology were at the low end of normal. These factors could have been contributing to the difficulty this couple was experiencing in getting pregnant. Fortunately, there were things that could help get Jack's swimmers back on track.

Jack and his partner were thrilled to have this additional level of information. Jack now understood that "normal" *does not* mean "optimal" and how big of a role the sperm factor played in their ability to get pregnant. Our plan was to incorporate a few simple natural lifestyle changes he could make to help improve his sperm.

The course of action we put in place to support Jack's fertility and overall health will be shared throughout future chapters of this book and will highlight how seemingly small modifications can make a big impact on sperm health.

To Test or Not to Test Sperm

There are no hard-and-fast rules for fertility testing and analysis from a timing perspective. I often see clients falling into one of two camps when it comes to testing: Either they want to test immediately (knowledge is power!) or they are reluctant to test (what if something is wrong?).

I am all for data (as you could probably guess!), but I also like to balance it with practicality. If you are at the beginning of your journey to parenthood, you don't need to rush out and order a semen analysis or DNA fragmentation testing. You are reading this book at the perfect time! All of the strategies in this book will help you build a strong foundation for healthy sperm and fertility. Remember, it takes about 2 months for changes to affect the sperm that is released, so take some time to incorporate these strategies and know you are building long-term health habits as well.

If you've been at it for a few months with no success, a general rule is:

- If one partner is getting tested (typically day 3 blood work for ovulating people), then both partners should test, starting with a semen analysis.

- If you are using a donor egg, then I recommend testing at the beginning of the process so you don't waste time or money if there is a problem.

- If you have been trying to get pregnant for 4–6 months without success, it's time to test.

- If you have experienced two or more miscarriages, it's time to test.

- If the sperm-producing partner is over 40 years old, consider testing.

- If you feel that there may be a problem (past illness, genetics, or even gut instinct), it is completely reasonable to seek out testing.

My recommendation is to start with a semen analysis before considering advanced testing. Most primary care doctors will order a semen analysis at your request. Just keep in mind Jack's story: Normal does not mean optimal. And now that you know how to navigate a semen analysis report, you can make an informed decision on the next steps to take.

The other piece of the testing puzzle to keep in mind is the emotional side. Testing can bring up all kinds of feelings and questions: What if something is wrong, what if this is all "my fault," what if I can't have a biological child, what impact will this have on our relationship? These are common reactions and something to discuss with your partner, a counselor, and/or your doctor. However, they are not reasons to avoid testing. I promise that facing any potential issues early in your fertility journey is worth the discomfort around testing.

Getting a semen analysis can feel scary, and awkward, but it is an important first step in the path to parenthood. Most importantly, if you are worried about the results of your testing, be assured that the strategies in this book are a collection of science-backed interventions to help improve sperm parameters and your chances of becoming pregnant. There are steps you can take to resolve issues uncovered through testing.

The bottom line is sperm won't fix themselves, and the sooner you start the sooner you can expect results.

CHAPTER 6

FUELING FERTILITY
WITH NUTRITION

·······························

How a Balanced Diet Sets the Stage for Egg and Sperm Health

Perhaps I am stating the obvious here, but good nutrition is as critical for optimal fertility as it is for overall health. Giving your body the right nourishment provides the ideal quantity of nutrients needed for egg and sperm development and hormone balance. Before we discuss herbs and supplements to help support a holistic fertility plan, it's important to build a strong foundation in nutrition. Herbs and supplements are not substitutes for a healthy diet.

Eating to Support Fertility

Supporting optimal fertility means eating a variety of unprocessed, whole foods with plenty of veggies. This isn't about restricting, or eating less, but adding the *right foods* to fuel your fertility. Fertility-boosting foods are high in antioxidants and include a combination of healthy fats, proteins, and fiber at every snack and meal.

So what is the best diet for fertility? Let me just be clear: By "diet" I *do not* mean weight loss. I am referring to the different foods you consume and which ones will best support your fertility journey.

The topic of nutrition is controversial, with a wide range of opinions. Even among nutritionists you will find varying recommendations influenced by personal experiences, philosophical perspectives, and specialized areas of expertise. Nutrition research frequently finds conflicting results, with certain diets showing success in some studies but not in others. Sometimes eating foods perceived as "healthy" may not necessarily be supportive to fertility.

Although a universally ideal diet may not exist, research-backed guidelines provide valuable insights into the foods that best support your run-up to pregnancy and can be grouped into three categories: nutrient-dense foods, blood sugar–balancing meals and snacks, and foods that support gut health.

Nutrient-Dense Foods

The processes of egg development, ovulation, maintaining regular menstrual cycles, and sperm production demand a significant amount of nutrients. Unfortunately, many of us fall short of meeting these demands. In fact, nutrient deficiencies are more common than you may realize, with nearly 30 percent of US adults being at risk for having at least one deficiency.[1] This trend is likely exacerbated by the fact that our fruits, vegetables, and grains contain fewer nutrients than they did a generation ago.

NUTRIENTS THAT SUPPORT FERTILITY

Taking deliberate steps to supercharge your diet with a diverse array of nutrient-rich foods becomes crucial in laying the foundation for nourishing fertility. Let's start at the beginning by first asking the questions: What nutrients are we talking about, and what roles do they play on your journey to conception? Here's a quick peek under the hood.

- **Choline:** supports ovarian function and egg and sperm quality

- **Iron:** supports ovulation

- **Lycopene:** protects sperm from oxidative stress and improves their quality

- **Magnesium:** maintains a good blood supply to the uterus, is needed for progesterone, helps decrease inflammation, and supports sperm quality

- **Manganese:** supports ovulation

- **Selenium:** critical for sperm quality and supports healthy egg development

- **Vitamin A:** supports egg and sperm quality, cervical fluid, and embryo implantation

- **Vitamin B_1 (thiamin):** necessary for healthy eggs, regular ovulation, and normal testicular function

- **Vitamin B_2 (riboflavin):** supports sperm and egg quality

- **Vitamin B_6 (pyridoxine):** aids in increasing cervical mucus, supporting progesterone levels, and preparing the uterine lining for implantation

- **Vitamin B_9 (folate):** supports egg quality, ovulation, and sperm quality, and increases pregnancy rates

- **Vitamin B_{12}:** facilitates the development and release of eggs for ovulation, supports sperm quality, and prevents DNA damage in sperm cells

- **Vitamin C:** improves sperm quality, decreases sperm DNA fragmentation, and supports follicular development and ovulation

- **Vitamin D:** associated with higher pregnancy rates and decreased miscarriage rates

- **Vitamin E**: enhances the lining of the uterus and increases the sperm's ability to penetrate an egg

- **Vitamin K:** helps the body effectively absorb nutrients and maintain hormonal balance

- **Zinc:** necessary for a regular menstrual cycle and development of healthy eggs, supports healthy testosterone production and sperm quality, and is needed for embryo implantation

And this is just the tip of the iceberg! Remember, the number of things that need to happen for egg and sperm development, ovulation, fertilization, implantation, and development of a healthy baby is truly astounding. Ensuring your body receives the necessary nutrients from a diverse diet of whole foods is essential for this process to happen.

You may think that because you are eating a "healthy" diet, full of good stuff and not so much bad stuff, you can skip this section. The key is in the *density* of the nutrients, and this is where you should focus. The easiest way to eat more nutrient-dense foods is to reduce processed foods and replace them with whole foods.

DOES WEIGHT MATTER FOR FERTILITY?

Research shows that weight can affect fertility.[2] Hormones play an important role in fertility, and being underweight or overweight can throw off your hormones, which can impact periods, ovulation, and sperm production. How do you know if your weight is in a healthy range for fertility? Start by calculating your body mass index (BMI) (search "BMI calculator" on the internet). Studies show that your best chance of getting pregnant is if your BMI is between 19 and 24 for the ovulating partner and between 20 and 25 for the sperm-producing partner. Following the guidelines in this book will help support a healthy BMI.

FOODS THAT MAKE UP A NUTRIENT-DENSE DIET

The next question is, invariably: How do I get these nutrients into my system? The answer is easier than you may think.

- **Veggies:** six to eight servings daily—kale, spinach, Swiss chard, collard greens, broccoli, bok choy, cauliflower, Brussels sprouts, bell peppers, tomatoes, beets, squash, sweet potatoes
- **Fruits:** two to three servings daily—berries, citrus fruits, pomegranates, avocados
- **Low-mercury fish:** two or three times per week—salmon, anchovies, herring, mackerel, sardines, shrimp, tilapia, cod
- **Eggs:** organic, pasture-raised (don't skip the yolk—that's where all the nutrients are!)
- **Meat or chicken:** organic, pasture-raised, grass-fed
- **Legumes:** chickpeas, lentils, beans
- **Nuts and seeds:** almonds, walnuts, Brazil nuts, pumpkin seeds, flaxseeds, chia seeds
- **Fermented foods:** sauerkraut, kimchi
- **Whole grains:** quinoa, amaranth, oats
- **Herbal tea:** 1–4 cups per day (see Chapter 8 for some of my favorites)
- **Herbs and spices:** generous use

When possible, choose organic to help reduce exposure to pesticides, and locally grown or locally raised foods because the shorter the time between harvest and when it lands on your table means it is less likely the nutrient value has decreased.

EVERY SMALL STEP COUNTS

I find that most people know they *should* be eating more nutrient-dense foods, especially vegetables, but they struggle to make it happen. First and foremost, know that every small step you make is moving your health in the right direction! This isn't an all-or-nothing approach, and perfection doesn't exist. Working with a qualified practitioner or coach can help take the things you know you should do and translate them into healthy habits.

The tips throughout this chapter will help you start making significant changes in the nutrient density of your daily diet, as will Chapter 8 (Herbs for Everyone). It's easier than you think; even enjoying a cup (or three!) of herbal tea daily will boost your intake of antioxidants and phytonutrients.

WHAT COUNTS AS A SERVING?

- Raw, leafy vegetables: 1 cup
- Cooked green, orange, or yellow veggies: ½ cup
- Tomatoes: 1 medium
- Avocados: ¼ of the avocado
- Potatoes and sweet potatoes: 1 cup
- Whole fruit, medium size (apple, banana): 1
- Berries: ½ cup

Blood Sugar-Balancing Meals and Snacks

While most of us know sugar isn't the healthiest choice, the specific reasons for its negative effects on hormone balance, fertility, and pregnancy often are less understood. Eating sugar, and carbohydrates in general, leads to fluctuations in blood sugar levels, characterized by spikes and subsequent drops. The more pronounced these fluctuations, the greater the negative impact on overall health and fertility (it doesn't feel very good either!). The goal is to minimize these rapid spikes and dramatic dips for a more balanced and stable blood sugar level.

Blood sugar fluctuations act as a form of stress on the body, raising levels of the stress hormone cortisol, which can interfere with reproductive hormones (more on stress and fertility in Chapter 9). Studies have also linked elevated blood sugar to decreased egg quality and increased levels of sperm DNA damage.

While it might come across as yet another fertility hack, learning how to eat for blood sugar balance is so much more. It's a skill that can transform your daily well-being and long-term health. Maintaining blood sugar balance is the key to steady energy, reducing insistent food cravings, keeping your mood on an even keel, ensuring hormonal balance, enhancing sleep quality, preventing chronic diseases, and creating an optimal setting for fertility.

WHAT ARE CARBOHYDRATES?

Despite their sometimes negative reputation, carbohydrates are essential for fueling the body. Not all carbs are equal, but carbs are crucial nutrients that your body converts into glucose, providing the energy needed for optimal function.

There are three main types of carbohydrates.

- Sugar: found naturally in some fruits, vegetables, and dairy, or added to foods such as cookies, sugary drinks, and candy

- Starch: found in some vegetables, grains, and beans

- Fiber: found in some fruits, vegetables, whole grains, and beans

All carbs can be classified as either a simple or a complex carbohydrate.

Simple carbohydrates are digested quickly and send immediate bursts of glucose into the bloodstream. Examples are milk, fruit juice, table sugar, candy, and baked goods.

Complex carbohydrates are digested more slowly and supply a slower release of glucose into the bloodstream. Examples are bread, rice, fiber-rich fruits and veggies, beans, lentils, quinoa, oats, and chia seeds. Fruits and vegetables are technically composed of simple carbohydrates, but their fiber, protein, and additional nutrients make them function more like complex carbohydrates within the body.

For the most part, fibers and starches are complex carbs, while sugars are simple carbs.

Although it is generally accepted that it's healthier to eat more complex carbs, all carbs are useful to our bodies. In the end, it's about balance and moderation.

HOW BLOOD SUGAR WORKS IN THE BODY

Every cell in the body needs energy—preferably from glucose—to survive. The main way to get glucose is by eating carbohydrates, either simple or complex. When you eat any type of carbohydrate, the body breaks it down into glucose, which is absorbed into the blood. Insulin is then released to help move this glucose from the bloodstream into the cells, so it can be used for energy. Insulin also helps store unused glucose in the liver for later use. Simple carbohydrates are digested quickly and spike blood sugar faster and higher. Complex carbohydrates are digested more slowly and release glucose into the bloodstream gradually. Overall, the slower the better.

This doesn't mean that all simple carbs are bad, or that you should never eat simple carbs. It just means you have to pair your carbs with healthy fats, protein, and fiber to help slow the release of glucose to smooth out the spikes and dips.

THREE SIGNS YOU'RE RIDING THE BLOOD SUGAR ROLLER COASTER

- Food cravings: constantly yearning for something sweet or high in carbs

- Frequently hungry: feeling the need to eat every couple of hours

- Fatigue: experiencing sudden exhaustion, where the idea of curling up for a nap seems like the best thing ever

Remember, how you feel is directly tied to the spikes and dips in your glucose levels. Smooth out those highs and lows, and you're on the path to feeling your absolute best!

HOW TO EAT FOR BLOOD SUGAR BALANCE

The secret to blood sugar balance is making sure every meal and snack has adequate protein, fat, and fiber. Never eat a carbohydrate on its own. Instead of an apple, have apple slices with almond butter. If you want to have a piece of toast, add avocado and smoked salmon. Over time, this will feel like second nature as you enjoy feeling more energized, stay full longer, and crave fewer sweets. For those of you who like numbers, here are some guidelines to help get you started.

- Each meal: 25–30 g of protein, 7–10 g of fiber, 3–7 g of fat, 30–45 g of carbohydrates

- Daily: approximately 100 g of protein, 30–35 g of fiber, 10–20 g of fat, 90–150 g of carbohydrates

Remember to listen to your body and notice how you feel after each meal. Some people feel great with meals that have 15–20 g of protein, while others need 30–40 g to feel satiated. You may find you need more protein if you are working out more and building muscle. Trust yourself over following a strict protocol.

PROTEIN BY THE SOURCE

Understanding the protein content of various sources can help you make informed choices. People often misjudge their total protein intake, so tracking for a few days can be quite eye-opening. Here's a quick guide of the protein amounts in common animal and plant proteins.

Animal Protein per Serving

A serving size is about 3½ ounces, unless otherwise indicated below. Each serving contains the following amount of protein.

Chicken breast, skinless: 32 g

Turkey breast, skinless, roasted: 30 g

Beef roast: 28 g

Pork roast: 27 g

Ground beef: 26 g

Tilapia: 26 g

Salmon: 25 g

Halibut: 23 g

Canned tuna, light, in water: 19 g

Shrimp: 17 g

Eggs: 12 g (or 6 g per egg)

Whole-milk Greek yogurt (⅓ cup): 9 g

Plant Protein per Serving

A serving size is about 3½ ounces, unless otherwise indicated below. Each serving contains the following amount of protein.

Kidney beans: 30 g

Lentils: 25 g

Black beans: 21 g

Plant-based protein powder: typically 20 g per serving

Tempeh: 20 g

Edamame: 12 g

Spirulina (3 tablespoons): 12 g

Hemp seeds (3 tablespoons): 9 g

Tofu: 9 g

Chickpeas, canned, drained: 8 g

Almonds (handful, about 23): 6 g

Almond butter (1 tablespoon): 3 g

STRATEGIES TO STOP THE BLOOD SUGAR ROLLER COASTER

Swap out the carb-heavy or sweet breakfast for a protein-packed, savory option. Your breakfast choice sets the tone for the entire day. Opting for a bowl of oatmeal with brown sugar and a banana may sound healthy, but it's heavy on carbs and will give you an initial glucose spike, swiftly followed by a sharp dip, leaving you hungry, fatigued, grumpy, and clouded with brain fog. By adding 2 tablespoons of nut butter, swapping the banana for berries, and adding a hard-boiled egg on the side, you can shift to a more balanced blood sugar level. Aim for 30–50 g of protein at breakfast. Here's a good example: three organic, pasture-raised eggs; two chicken sausage links; and ½ of an avocado served over a cup of arugula with a handful of raspberries on the side. That's a breakfast that will keep you feeling energized and satiated for hours.

EMBRACE THE PLATE METHOD

Ditch the pyramid and embrace the plate—a more balanced approach to meals. The plate method is an easy, visual way to plan out your meals without measuring or weighing portions. Fill half of your plate (about 2 cups) with nonstarchy vegetables (broccoli, carrots, cauliflower, asparagus, Brussels sprouts, cabbage, mushrooms, peppers, leafy greens), a quarter of your plate (3–4 ounces) with protein (eggs, fish, meat, seafood, tempeh, tofu), and the remainder of your plate with carbohydrate-rich whole foods (grains, beans, legumes, starchy vegetables such as sweet potatoes or squash). Make sure you have 1–2 tablespoons of healthy fat as part of your protein (chicken with the skin on or fatty fish, olive oil, nuts, seeds, avocado, butter, ghee, coconut milk).

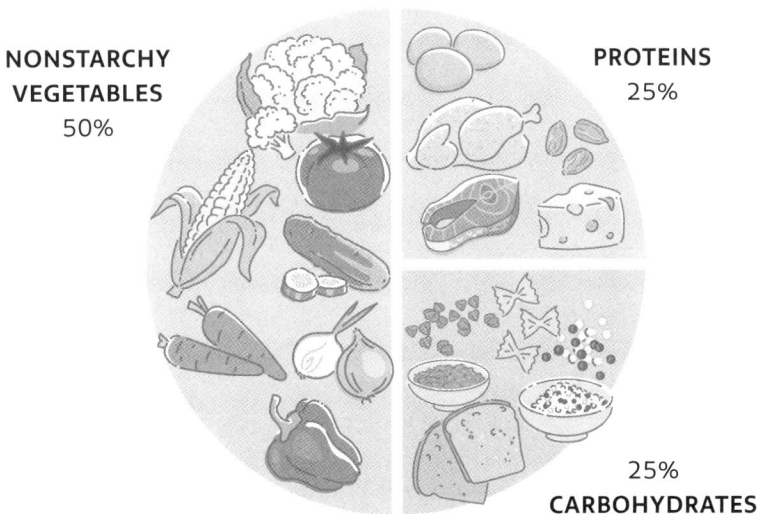

NONSTARCHY VEGETABLES 50%

PROTEINS 25%

25% CARBOHYDRATES

ENJOY BLOOD SUGAR–BALANCING SNACKS

Snack if you need to, but always with a blood sugar–balancing combination. Remember, no carbohydrates without protein, fiber, and fat! Some examples:

- A handful of almonds with berries and dark chocolate

- Nut butter protein balls (see Chapter 8 for recipe)

- Cucumber slices with avocado and smoked salmon

- Hummus with veggies and kalamata olives

- Guacamole with veggies

- Chia seed pudding with almonds and berries

- Whole-grain toast with avocado and tomato slices

- Hard-boiled egg with berries

- Trail mix with nuts, seeds, and dark chocolate

- Smoothie balanced with protein and fat

Almond Cinnamon Balanced Smoothie

This delicious smoothie includes protein, fats, and carbs, balanced in a way that won't spike your blood sugar.

1¼   cups unsweetened almond milk
1   scoop protein powder
1   tablespoon ground flaxseed
1   tablespoon almond butter
½   avocado
1   teaspoon ground cinnamon
     Handful of ice (optional)

Place the ingredients in a blender and blend.

SKIP THE JUICE

Yes, even the fresh-pressed, organic, gourmet juice. Fruit, when juiced, loses its fiber, so it's pure fructose and will result in a rapid, sharp glucose spike. Of course, you can choose to indulge in the occasional glass, but only as a special treat and be ready for that glucose spike and drop, as you would with a piece of cake or other dessert! Smoothies with fruits in them can also be a problem, but can be balanced by adding—you guessed it—more fat and protein! So a smoothie with some berries, spinach, almond butter, avocado, and protein powder is better than a strawberry, banana, spinach smoothie. It's better to eat whole fruit.

EMBRACE HEALTHY FATS

Healthy fats nourish our bodies and fertility. Scientific research has debunked the myths that fats are universally bad and that anything labeled "low-fat" equates to health. It's important to note that not all fats are created equal. Your best course of action is to opt for high-quality sources like these:

- Butter or ghee
- Coconut oil, extra-virgin olive oil, avocado oil
- Nuts and seeds (and oil from nuts and seeds)
- Avocados, olives
- Fats found in chicken, beef, fish, and eggs

Foods That Support Gut Health

Your body is home to a community of trillions of microorganisms, including 38 trillion bacteria (yes, that's *trillion*). Your microbiome is made up of these tiny, living organisms and everything that exists around them in a particular area of your body. While the most well-known microbiome is the gut, the body has several, including oral, skin, vaginal, uterine, prostate, and seminal microbiomes, each with their very own unique diversity of microorganisms.

The various microbiomes in the body contribute to important daily functions, such as stimulating the immune system, reducing inflammation, synthesizing vitamins, and influencing mood, appetite, behavior, and circadian rhythm. Research has found a strong connection between the microbiome and fertility. Did you know:

- The semen microbiome affects sperm development and motility.[3]

- The vaginal microbiome can influence the success of IVF procedures, with specific microbial profiles associated with improved implantation and pregnancy rates.[4]

- The gut microbiome affects testosterone production and egg development, regulates insulin, and contributes to inflammation and obesity, all of which play a role in fertility.[5]

- The gut microbiome can regulate sleep, improve mood, and improve resilience to developing anxiety or depression when under stress, all of which are important when trying to get pregnant.[6,7]

Research is still emerging, but it suggests the different microbiomes of the body work together to support fertility and, over time, may provide more clues to resolving unexplained infertility.

CAN THE PILL HURT YOUR MICROBIOME?

If you have been taking oral contraceptive pills (OCPs or "the pill"), you may need to give your microbiome a little extra love. OCPs can disrupt both the vaginal and the gut microbiome. Studies have shown that OCPs can negatively impact gut flora and estrogen metabolism, and OCPs increase the incidence of vaginal yeast infections.[8,9] Irritable bowel syndrome, gas, bloating, constipation, acne, and eczema can all be signs of an imbalanced microbiome or dysbiosis.

HOW TO SUPPORT YOUR MICROBIOME

Your microbiome is established during birth and over the first 2 years of life. It will continue to change over your lifetime, influenced by foods, drinks, medications, illnesses, stress, and environmental exposures. It is a living, dynamic, and fast-changing environment, with some microbes living only 20 minutes. When the balance of beneficial and harmful microorganisms in the microbiome is disturbed and not rebalanced, it results in microbiome dysbiosis.

Now for the good news! You have tremendous influence over your microbiome and, within just a few weeks, can begin to rebalance your system through what you eat and drink. A diverse and balanced diet, promoting the growth of beneficial bacteria while discouraging the problematic bacteria, creates a healthy environment for the microbiome.

Here are some tips to help your microbiome thrive:

Eat more probiotic foods. Probiotic foods contain live, beneficial bacteria. Consuming these foods daily improves the microbiome by directly increasing the numbers of beneficial bacteria in your gut.

Examples of probiotic foods include yogurt, kefir, kimchi, miso, tempeh, sauerkraut, and unpasteurized, fermented pickles. (Pro tip: Check the label; if *vinegar* or *pasteurized* is indicated on the label, it doesn't contain probiotics.)

Improving your microbiome through foods is easier than you might think. Whether it's a spoonful of sauerkraut, a serving of fermented pickles as a flavorful side dish, or infusing a salad with the zesty kick of kimchi, these simple additions help introduce beneficial bacteria and can have a big impact. Just 1 tablespoon of sauerkraut provides between 10 million and 10 billion colony forming units (CFUs), and one fermented pickle contains between 1 billion and 18 billion CFUs (depending on the batch). For comparison, most probiotic supplements contain between 10 billion and 50 billion CFUs. Enhancing the microbiome through dietary choices can take anywhere from a few days to several weeks. Even if changes aren't noticeable, trust that the microbiome is slowly rebalancing and don't give up.

Eat more prebiotic food. *Pre*biotic foods are nondigestible plant fibers that feed the beneficial gut bacteria. While *pro*biotics introduce good bacteria into the gut, *pre*biotics are the food good bacteria eat. They help our good bacteria thrive and grow.

Some examples of prebiotic foods are asparagus, Brussels sprouts, onions, leeks, peas, carrots, garlic, chicory root, dandelion greens, Jerusalem artichokes, mushrooms, underripe bananas, jicama, flaxseeds, legumes, barley, oats, and apples. Try to consume a few of these whole foods each day.

Incorporate herbal bitters before meals. Herbal bitters are a type of liquid extract made from bitter herbs. Bitters play a crucial role in balancing stomach acid secretion and bile release and are essential for breaking down food and absorbing fats and vital nutrients.

Add a healthy dose of bitters to your diet every day, either as an herbal tincture (more on herbal tinctures in Chapter 8) taken before a meal or by adding bitter herbs to foods, using things like dandelion greens, burdock root, arugula, kale, and ginger.

Eat less sugar. While prebiotic fiber is what the good bacteria feeds on, sugar is food for the bad guys. When these undesirable microbes thrive, they can outnumber the beneficial bacteria, leading to dysbiosis. This sets off a cycle of sugar cravings, as the undesirable bacteria send signals to the brain, prompting more sugar cravings.

You don't have to eliminate all sugars; moderation is key. Even a simple switch in sweeteners can help; for example, honey and dark chocolate (with at least 70 percent cocoa) are great prebiotics and have loads of extra health benefits.

WHAT ABOUT ARTIFICIAL SWEETENERS?

Artificial sweeteners like saccharin, sucralose, and aspartame also have a negative effect on the gut and oral microbiomes. When consumed for as little as 2 weeks, these sweeteners have a significant negative effect, with some reducing the body's ability to regulate blood glucose levels, leading to weight gain and diabetes.[10] So drop that packet and try honey, maple sugar, or just less regular sugar.

MORE WAYS TO SUPPORT YOUR MICROBIOME

Get dirty in the garden. Soil is full of beneficial microorganisms, including bacteria, that support our microbiome. Digging in the soil, pulling weeds, planting seeds, and harvesting vegetables all put us into direct contact with the soil and its diverse microorganisms. Those microorganisms can make their way into our body, supporting our microbiome. So skip the gloves and get your hands dirty.

Get a furry pet. Homes with dogs, cats, and other furry pets have greater beneficial bacterial diversity than pet-free homes do. As we are exposed to these bacteria, they work their way onto and into our bodies. Studies with infants and young children have shown that early life exposure to household pets increases richness and diversity of the children's microbiome,[11] not to mention the added benefit having wonderful companions.

Manage stress. The connection between our gut and our brain is a two-way street. A healthy microbiome produces feel-good neurotransmitters like serotonin and dopamine. When we are stressed, the brain sends signals to the gut that trigger unfavorable shifts in bacterial composition and diversity. Don't let stress overwhelm you! In Chapter 9, you'll find a variety of strategies to help you navigate and manage stress effectively.

Avoid NSAIDs when possible. Nonsteroidal anti-inflammatory drugs (NSAIDs) such as aspirin and ibuprofen can be hard on the digestive system as a whole, but in particular on the gut lining and gut microbiome. Studies have shown that just one dose of NSAIDs was capable of changing the balance of bacteria in the digestive tract, and people who took NSAIDs regularly had significant differences in the composition of their gut bacteria.

Don't douche. The vagina is a self-cleansing organ, and douching can do more harm than good. Douching can increase the risks of bacterial vaginosis, preterm birth, and pelvic inflammatory disease and decrease the presence of *Lactobacillus* (the beneficial bacteria associated with improved IVF embryo implantation rates).

Fueling your body for fertility has long-lasting health advantages. By prioritizing nutrient-dense foods, maintaining balanced blood sugar levels, and supporting your microbiome, you not only enhance fertility but significantly lower the risk of chronic diseases. Incorporate small, consistent steps into your daily routine, and with time, nourishing your body for fertility will become a natural and sustainable practice.

Foods to Avoid or Reduce

Now that you have a plan to help fuel your fertility, let's dive into the stuff to steer clear of (or at least cut back on). These foods lack nutritional value, may negatively affect your chances of conception, and could pose other health risks.

Trans Fats

Trans fats are bad for your health and detrimental to your fertility. They can decrease sperm count and quality, negatively affect egg quality, and increase the risk of developing ovulatory infertility.[12]

Studies have shown that even small amounts of trans fats in the diet can have a negative impact on fertility. People who consumed 2 percent of their daily calories in the form of trans fats (which translates to 4 g for a person eating 1,800 calories a day) exhibited an average of a 76 percent greater chance of developing ovulatory infertility.[13]

Trans fats are made when liquid oils are turned into solid fats, like shortening or margarine. These are called partially hydrogenated oils and are found in fried foods, packaged snacks, commercial baked goods, and other sources. Although trans fats have been banned in the United States since 2020, it can be tricky to completely avoid them. In the United States, manufacturers can label their products "trans-fat-free" as long as there are fewer than 0.5 g per serving. While 0.5 g may sound like a tiny amount, if you eat more than one serving, or if it's a food you eat regularly, it can add up quickly. To completely eliminate trans fats from the diet, read the labels and steer clear of foods listing hydrogenated or partially hydrogenated oils in their ingredients.

Here are some sneaky sources of trans fats to avoid.

- Commercial baked goods, such as cakes, cookies, and pies
- Shortening
- Microwave popcorn
- Frozen pizza
- Refrigerated dough, such as biscuits and rolls
- Fried foods, including french fries, doughnuts, and fried chicken
- Nondairy coffee creamer
- Margarine

Industrial Seed Oils

Industrial seed oils, also called vegetable oils, are highly processed oils like canola, corn, and soybean oils. Unlike traditional fats, such as olive oil, coconut oil, butter, and ghee, industrial seed oils are a recent addition to the human diet that are devoid of nutrients, are calorically dense, and don't support your fertility.

These oils are rich in *pro*-inflammatory omega-6 fats, contributing to chronic inflammation that can disrupt hormone production and affect conception and implantation processes. Additionally, industrial seed oils can form free radicals and reactive oxygen species that generate oxidative stress in the body. As discussed in Chapters 2 and 3, oxidative stress is bad for egg and sperm development.

Commonly used in restaurants, especially for deep-frying, these oils also sneak into foods marketed as "healthy," like whole-grain crackers, protein bars, dressings, and even some frozen foods and chocolates.

Always read labels and avoid the following oils:

- Canola (aka rapeseed oil)
- Soybean
- Corn
- Safflower
- Sunflower
- Cottonseed
- Grapeseed
- Rice bran
- Peanut

Opt for healthier alternatives like extra-virgin olive oil, avocado oil, coconut oil, and grass-fed butter or ghee for fertility-friendly choices.

Soda

Daily soda consumption may jeopardize your chances of conceiving. Research has shown that when an ovulating partner drank one sugar-sweetened soda daily, they experienced a 25 percent lower chance of pregnancy, and this jumped to 52 percent when they consumed three servings per day.[14] Soda has an impact on sperm, too—just one serving per day decreased the chance of pregnancy by 33 percent.[15] It's believed that sugar-sweetened soda increases insulin resistance, leading to oxidative stress, which affects both semen quality and ovulatory function.

Considering a switch to diet soda? Unfortunately, the outlook on artificial sweeteners and fertility is not promising. A study on IVF patients showed that drinking any amount of diet soda negatively affected egg and embryo quality and reduced the chance of becoming pregnant.[16]

Alcohol

While the occasional drink is not likely to make an impact, moderate consumption of alcohol daily can significantly increase the risk of infertility. Excessive alcohol is linked to decreased ovarian reserve, lower testosterone, and decreased sperm parameters. Alcohol also contains sugar, which can affect blood sugar balance, disrupt the gut biome, and impact sleep, all of which are important for fertility. Limiting alcohol to one to two servings per week, or less, is best. It is also a good idea to avoid alcohol during the period of time when you think you could be pregnant (the weeks after ovulation and before your expected period) and continue abstaining once pregnant.

IVF AND ALCOHOL

For those undergoing IVF, even low alcohol consumption is believed to have a negative impact, by reducing egg quantity and resulting in lower pregnancy rates. To optimize the chances of successful fertility treatments, it is best to abstain from alcohol within 1 month of undergoing fertility treatment. If you are providing a sperm sample for IVF, it is recommended to avoid alcohol for at least 1 week before the procedure.

Excess Coffee

Good news: You don't have to give up your morning cup of joe! Most studies suggest that 12 ounces (or 200 mg) of caffeine per day is safe and shows no changes in fertility or increased risk of miscarriage, but more can be an issue.

One study showed that women who drank five or more cups of coffee a day severely reduced their chance of success from IVF treatment.[17] Researchers described the adverse impact as "comparable to the detrimental effect of smoking."

So don't drink five cups of coffee per day when you are trying to get pregnant (or ever, really). Switching out your morning coffee for green tea will help decrease your daily caffeine intake and help boost your daily antioxidant intake. Bonus: Antioxidants can help support egg and sperm quality.

The recommendations in this chapter will help you fuel your fertility and improve your health overall. Remember that it is all about balance, and you don't have to do everything perfectly all the time or all at once. Focus on small improvements over time . . . it will make a big difference!

JACK AND EMILY'S STORIES
A Nutritional Plan to Boost Fertility

When I met with Jack and his partner, they were focused on Jack's sperm parameters, which were on the very low end of normal. Before jumping into herbs and supplements to support Jack's sperm health, it was important to create a strong nutritional foundation and eliminate any common fertility saboteurs.

ANALYZING JACK'S FOOD DIARY

After a brief analysis of Jack's food diary, we noted that he consumed one to two servings of vegetables daily and just one serving of fruits. Jack's pattern was not uncommon, as most North Americans typically include only three servings of fruits and vegetables in their daily diet. Sperm require a lot of nutrients to develop optimally, so bumping up Jack's intake of veggies was a top priority. We also discovered that several of Jack's grab-and-go breakfast bars contained industrial seed oils and hydrogenated oils (trans fats)—all things to avoid for optimal sperm health.

JACK'S PLAN

Goal. Two servings of greens at each meal. This can be easier than you may think! For example:

Breakfast. One cup leftover roasted veggies, 2 eggs, ¼ of an avocado, 1 precooked piece of apple chicken sausage. That's three servings of veggies (yes, avocados are technically a fruit, but ¼ of an avocado counts as a serving of veggies!).

Lunch. Protein bowl: ½ cup quinoa, 1 cup greens (kale, arugula, mixed greens), 1 cup protein of choice (salmon, chicken, steak, chickpeas, tofu), ½ cup shelled edamame, dressing of choice (if store-bought, check the ingredient list for industrial seed or hydrogenated oils—olive oil, fresh lemon juice, and some Dijon mustard is a quick, healthy alternative to store-bought). Feel free to add more veggies as inspired: peppers, cucumbers, a handful of fresh herbs . . . have fun! That's another two (or more) servings of veggies.

Dinner. Protein and veggies. Roast a variety of veggies on cookie sheets while you are grilling up your favorite protein. Some favorites: Brussels sprouts, broccoli, cauliflower, sweet potatoes, asparagus, onions, kale, and zucchini. One-half cup of roasted veggies counts as a serving, so you can easily add one to two servings at dinner. Bonus: Cook enough so you have leftovers for breakfasts and lunches.

Snacks. A serving of fruit with nuts or nut butter, herbal nut balls (see Chapter 8), trail mix, or smoothies with protein and fats.

EMILY'S PRIORITIES

When we first met Emily in Chapter 2, she was concerned her age was affecting her fertility. She was motivated to do everything possible to support her egg quality, and while there are many herbs and supplements to consider, we first needed to ensure she had a strong foundation of nutrition and balanced blood sugar. A secondary focus for Emily was her painful menstrual cramps, which often required ibuprofen to manage. We started rebuilding her microbiome through probiotic-rich foods and at the same time put a plan in place to reduce her cramps.

EMILY'S PLAN

Bump up the veggies! Most of us need to make a conscious effort to get more veggies, particularly greens, into our diets. Similar to Jack's recommendations, we focused on adding one to three servings of veggies at every meal to help Emily meet her daily goals.

Start the day with a high-protein breakfast. This helped Emily feel more satiated and make healthier food choices throughout the day. To set herself up for success, Emily made a batch of vegetable egg muffins on the weekend for a quick, grab-and-go breakfast during the week.

Give the microbiome some love. More fermented foods: a side serving of sauerkraut, kimchi, or fermented pickles, one or two times per day.

Decrease or eliminate ibuprofen. We incorporated ginger tea to help relieve menstrual cramps (more details on Emily's ginger tea in Chapter 8).

Limit the evening wine. While completely avoiding alcohol isn't necessary, being mindful of how much and when is a better approach. Limit alcohol to 1 glass of wine per week. Emily was excited to experiment with mocktails and herbal teas to help satisfy the desire for a postdinner drink. (Check out my favorite tea recipes in Chapter 8.)

CHAPTER 7

SORTING THROUGH
SUPPLEMENTS

···

What's Safe, Effective, and Worthwhile

Having the right nutrients is critical for both the egg
and the sperm when you're trying to conceive. But let's
face it, keeping up with a perfectly balanced diet all the
time can be tough, especially with modern eating habits.
When you add in stress, chemicals in the environment,
and processed foods, our bodies become drained of
the vitamins and minerals needed to make a baby.
Supplements can help fill the gap.

Supplements for Eggs, Ovulation, and Cycle Hormones

Supplements offer a convenient and reliable way to ensure the body receives and maintains optimal levels of these nutrients and to address any deficiencies. But not all supplements live up to their hype. The truth is, many supplements on the market are not backed by solid science. In fact, some can be downright useless or even harmful. Supplements aren't cheap either, so before you jump on the bandwagon and make the investment, it's crucial to do your homework. First and foremost, make sure they are safe. Second, they need to be helpful for your fertility journey. And third, make sure they are the highest quality.

Prenatal Multivitamin

The number one supplement for anyone trying to conceive is a high-quality pre-natal multivitamin. The ingredients help your body maintain the right levels of nutrients crucial for egg quality, maturation, fertilization, and implantation and play a vital role in combating oxidative stress.

While many people recognize the importance of the prenatal vitamin for supporting a baby's development during pregnancy, its potential to help you get pregnant in the first place is often overlooked. It's called *pre*natal for a reason! A comprehensive prenatal multivitamin can positively impact fertility, whether you're just starting out or facing challenges conceiving. That's why it's recom-mended to start taking a prenatal at least 4 months before trying to conceive, ideally even a year ahead.

When it comes to selecting a top-quality prenatal, be picky! You might think any prenatal with folic acid is sufficient, but the reality is, not all prenatals include the same nutrients at the same doses. Some even contain additives, fill-ers, and artificial colors that could potentially be harmful.

Let's start with what to avoid in a prenatal multivitamin. Read the fine print!

Avoid artificial colors. The first step in choosing a prenatal vitamin is to eliminate the ones containing artificial colors. Artificial colors offer no benefit, and research indicates they could even be harmful. They're used to make the supplements look more appealing. I don't know about you, but "pretty" isn't a requirement for the pills I swallow!

Research with pregnant animals found a link between artificial colors, hyperactivity, and changes in behavior in offspring,[1] and human studies have established a connection between children consuming artificial colors and nega-tive effects on their behavior and neurodevelopment.[2]

Artificial colors are listed on ingredient labels as Blue #1 and #2, Citrus Red #2, Red #40, Yellow #5 and #6, Green #3, and Red #3, FD&C Blue No. 1, FD&C Yellow No. 5 and 6, and FD&C Red No. 40, or artificial color.

There is no reason to settle for a supplement with any of these unnecessary ingredients when better options exist. Eliminating brands that contain artificial colors will help you quickly rule out the lower-quality supplements before you move on to the next step.

BRAND CHOICE AND WHERE YOU BUY MATTERS

While the Food and Drug Administration (FDA) regulates supplements in the United States, supplements have fewer safety requirements than pharmaceutical drugs. It's up to the manufacturers, not the FDA, to ensure safety standards are being met before putting a supplement on the shelves. Adulterated supplements are a growing concern, with over 700 found to contain unapproved pharmaceutical ingredients from 2007 to 2016.[3] To make informed choices, opt for reputable brands and stores, checking for certifications like USDA Organic or Non-GMO Project Verified, and third-party verifications like NSF, USP Verified, and ConsumerLab (CL). Beware of online third-party sellers, as counterfeits have been reported on online shopping websites.

The Ultimate Prenatal Supplement Plan

Just as you might tailor a recipe to your dietary needs and preferences, selecting a prenatal multivitamin may involve a bit of customizing. The following nutrients are all important pieces of your prenatal protocol, but they don't have to be all in one pill. Depending on your unique situation, you may choose to have it included in the prenatal multi or supplemented separately.

FOLATE OR FOLIC ACID

Regardless of your overall health and how well you eat, supplementing with folic acid is critical when planning to conceive. Folate, in the form of folic acid, not only supports egg quality and ovulation but also plays a vital role in preventing neural tube defects (NTDs), which are severe birth defects of the brain or spine.

Recommended prenatal dosage: 400 mcg of folic acid (equivalent to 667 mcg DFE)

FOLIC ACID OR METHYLATED FOLATE?

You may have heard that if you have an MTHFR variant, you should take a methylated form of folate (such as 5-MTHF). The theory is that people with this gene variant have difficulty converting folic acid to its active form in the body, but this gene variant has not been proven to affect folate levels in research. In fact, studies have shown that even if you have the MTHFR variant, your body can safely and effectively process folic acid.[4]

In theory, methylated forms should raise folate levels and provide similar benefits,[5] but their effectiveness in preventing neural tube defects (NTDs) hasn't been proven in studies. Methylated folate is the form many high-quality prenatal multivitamins contain. Some brands include both types, just to make sure they've got all angles covered.

To be clear, folic acid is the only type of folate proven to help prevent NTDs, but theoretically, methylated forms should offer similar protection.

While not common, there are cases where a person has difficulty tolerating one form or the other. If this is a problem for you, work with your healthcare provider to find a form that you can tolerate.

IRON

Healthy iron levels decrease your chance of unexplained infertility. It's also crucial to head into any pregnancy with good levels, and in order to do that, you need to have the right amount in the conception phase.

Iron is one you may want to consider supplementing separately. Some people need more than 27 mg per day, some less, and the recommended dosage can be difficult to tolerate, leading to constipation. Iron can also interfere with certain medications, and when combined with calcium can negatively impact its absorption. This is why you may choose to take a prenatal that doesn't include iron and supplement separately. Try experimenting with different forms and times of day to help manage constipation and reach optimal iron levels.

Recommended dosage: 27 mg of iron per day

VITAMIN D

Vitamin D is a superstar nutrient. From its role in supporting the immune system to supporting healthy bones and mood, this nutrient has hormone-like effects that are essential for reproductive health and general wellness. It is good for fertility, with optimal levels of vitamin D being associated with increased fertility rates and decreased miscarriage rates. Low vitamin D is associated with endometriosis, polycystic ovary syndrome, and uterine fibroids, all of which can negatively impact fertility. Here are some research highlights.

- Studies have shown improved pregnancy rates in people undergoing IVF who had sufficient vitamin D levels compared to those who were deficient or insufficient.[6]

- Donor egg recipients with a normal vitamin D level had higher pregnancy rates than did those with a low vitamin D level.[7]

- Sufficient preconception vitamin D levels are associated with a reduced risk of miscarriage.[8]

About 35 percent of adults in the United States are vitamin D deficient, with even more falling short of the ideal range. The best way to make an informed decision about supplementation is to have your vitamin D levels checked by your doctor. Vitamin D levels are influenced by body weight, skin tone, sun exposure, health status, and many other factors. I've seen many people in my practice supplement but remain deficient or have levels exceeding the recommended levels. So don't guess—test!

For most people, supplementing between 2,000 and 4,000 IU is the correct dose, and some people will need more or less. You will not know the proper dose unless you are tested.

Most labs in the United States use 30 ng/mL as the cutoff for normal (equivalent to 75 nmol/L internationally). However, studies suggest that levels between 30 and 50 ng/mL (or 75–125 nmol/L) may be more beneficial for fertility. The research on fertility doesn't support higher levels being better.

Recommended dosage: Until you've tested, you can safely take between 1,000 and 2,000 IUs. Once you've tested and know your precise levels, consult a professional to achieve or maintain optimal levels. Don't take more than 4,000 IU (100 mcg) daily without supervision from your doctor, and make sure you account for all supplement sources. If your levels are below 20 ng/mL, work with your doctor to bring your levels up quickly but safely.

OMEGA-3 FATTY ACIDS

Omega-3s have been found to aid fertility by reducing inflammation, boosting ovulation and hormone production, and positively affecting egg development. Once pregnancy is underway, fish oil supplementation supports the baby's brain and eye development.

There are three main types of omega-3 fatty acids: alpha-linolenic acid (ALA), eicosapentaenoic acid (EPA), and docosahexaenoic acid (DHA). EPA and DHA are most commonly found in seafood, while ALA is typically found in plant oils. While DHA has been singled out over the years for healthy brain development in babies, studies also suggest that all omega-3 fatty acids play an important role in fertility.

Here's a highlight of some of the research.

- People who took an omega-3 supplement were almost two times more likely to get pregnant on their own versus the people who didn't take the supplement.[9]

- Higher levels of omega-3 fatty acids are associated with improved egg quality and pregnancy rates in IVF cycles.[10]

- Omega-3s increase blood flow to the uterus and reduce inflammation in the body, both of which can help improve fertility.

Omega-3-rich foods include cold-water fatty fish (e.g., salmon, sardines, trout, mussels), pasture-raised eggs, pasture-raised meat, and organ meat. While it is possible to meet omega-3 requirements through food alone (aim for two to three servings of cold-water fish per week), many people will need to supplement.

Recommended dosage: An omega-3 supplement of 1 g per day with at least 200 mg from DHA is a good place to start. Choose a high-quality brand of fish oil, one that has been tested by an independent third-party such as ConsumerLab or USP.

*Note: If you are a vegetarian or vegan, algae oil is a good plant-based source of DHA.

CHOLINE

Choline is required for fetal brain development, placental function, and preventing neural tube defects. While choline can be obtained from food, many people's diets fall short, especially if you don't eat eggs.

Recommended dosage: 450 mg including intake from food. Some studies show higher levels may be beneficial.

Here are a few food sources of choline:

- 1 egg, including the yolk: 145 mg
- 3 ounces ground beef: 72 mg
- 3 ounces chicken breast: 72 mg
- ½ cup beans: 45 mg
- ½ cup broccoli: 30 mg
- ¼ cup almonds: 18 mg

Piecing Together the Core Supplements

Once you have considered each of these nutrients and decided how each will be part of your prenatal regimen, you can make brand choices more confidently. It's like piecing together a puzzle—one prenatal might have all the vitamin D you need, but it lacks choline. Another could offer both vitamin D and choline, but it has too much iron for your liking. Then there's the option that ticks all your boxes except for DHA. You opt for that one and pair it with a separate omega-3 supplement containing EPA and DHA. Voilà! You have crafted your ideal prenatal supplement support kit. If you're having trouble putting all the pieces together, work with your healthcare provider for extra support.

Warning: More is *not* better. Any vitamin or nutrient in too high a dose can be dangerous, particularly in pregnancy. To be on the safe side, steer clear of the upper limit (UL) dosage for any nutrient and be sure to take an inventory of all the supplements (including powders, smoothies, teas, and any other supplements) to be sure you aren't accidentally getting too much of a certain vitamin or nutrient.

Take only one serving of your prenatal multivitamin each day, based on what the recommended daily serving is as indicated on the label. If you need an extra amount of a vitamin or mineral, take it as a separate supplement.

Additional Supplements to Consider

While prenatal multivitamins lay a strong foundation for preconception health, additional supplements tailored to your individual needs can further support your fertility.

COENZYME Q10 (CoQ10)

You may recall from biology class that mitochondria are the cell's powerhouse because they generate most of the energy needed to power a cell's biochemical reactions. Did you know that egg cells have more mitochondria than any other cell in the body? These mitochondria are crucial for providing the energy needed to develop healthy eggs. That's where the antioxidant CoQ10 comes into play. CoQ10 is essential for energy production within the mitochondria; it supports cell functions by producing energy in the form of adenosine triphosphate and neutralizing free radicals. However, as we get older, CoQ10 levels naturally decline, which can affect egg quality. Studies show that CoQ10 supplementation can be beneficial in supporting fertility, especially for people over 35 and those who have diminished ovarian reserve.[11]

Use and dosage: CoQ10 is fat soluble, so it should be taken with a meal containing fat so your body can absorb it. Soft gels tend to be better absorbed than capsules or other preparations. Studies used doses ranging from 100 to 600 mg per day.

PROBIOTICS

The microbiome thrives best when we make healthy food choices every day, as highlighted in Chapter 6. However, there are times when taking a supplement is beneficial. For example, if you've had prolonged or frequent use of antibiotics, NSAIDs, or OCPs in the past, your microbiome may need extra support.

Use and dosage: On top of your daily dose of fermented foods, probiotic supplements can help balance the gut and vaginal microbiome. Look for an oral probiotic with at least 10 billion CFUs and a diversity of *Lactobacillus* and *Bifidobacterium* strains. If you have a history of vaginal yeast infections or bacterial vaginosis, choose a probiotic specifically formulated for vaginal health that includes *Lactobacillus rhamnosus* and *Lactobacillus reuteri*.

Between choosing your essential prenatal multivitamins and considering adding supplements like CoQ10 or probiotics, you'll likely cover all your bases for supporting fertility and early pregnancy. In Chapter 11, we'll delve into additional supplements to address common conditions that may affect your fertility.

WHAT'S THE BEST TIME OF DAY TO TAKE PRENATAL SUPPLEMENTS?

In general, you can take your prenatal supplements whenever it is most convenient for you, with the following considerations.

- Always take your prenatal multivitamin with food.

- If your prenatal multivitamin requires several capsules, you can divide your dosage and take multiple times throughout the day or take them all at once based on your preference.

- It's best to take your prenatal multivitamin separate from other medications and herbs to avoid any potential absorption issues.

- Calcium can affect how the body takes in the nutrients iron, zinc, and magnesium. The small amounts in prenatal multivitamins is likely not an issue, but if you choose to add a calcium supplement, take it 1–2 hours away from other supplements.

Supplements for Sperm

Preconception supplements aren't just for the egg! Sperm need nutrients to be healthy, too. The quality, movement, and shape of sperm are crucial for getting pregnant and a healthy pregnancy.

Multivitamin

The testes are always busy producing sperm, and they rely on specific resources to keep up the production. Antioxidants like CoQ10, vitamin C, vitamin E, lycopene, and selenium play a big role in keeping sperm healthy and improving the chances that your swimmers will reach their target and complete their mission. These antioxidants work by protecting sperm from free radicals, which are a significant factor in many cases of infertility.

Although it's ideal to get these essential nutrients from food, achieving optimal amounts can be challenging in our modern world. A multivitamin can bridge the gaps and address any deficiencies, ensuring your body can support the best possible sperm production.

Most high-quality multivitamins contain everything you need for making healthy sperm. Make sure you read the labels and look for a multivitamin that does not contain artificial colors and does contain the antioxidants mentioned above (CoQ10, vitamin C, vitamin E, lycopene, and selenium), plus nutrients such as carnitine, zinc, and folate.

OMEGA-3 FATTY ACIDS (FISH OIL)

Sperm cells contain high amounts of omega-3 and omega-6 fatty acids, which are required for optimal sperm cell flexibility and movement. DHA and EPA, two forms of omega-3s, help improve the sperm membranes and protect them from oxidative damage. DHA is necessary for binding the building blocks of a sperm's pointy cap, called the acrosome. This is crucial, since the acrosome contains the enzymes that allow the sperm to pierce the egg, causing fertilization.

Studies have found that people with higher omega-3 levels tend to have healthier sperm,[12] and even short-term supplementation of DHA and EPA over 10 weeks improves sperm concentration, motility, morphology, and DNA fragmentation.[13]

Use and dosage: Your body can't make omega-3 fats on its own, so we get them either from diet or through supplements. While eating fish a couple of times a week is a good start, many people need more. Taking a daily supplement containing a blend of DHA and EPA, typically 1.5–2 g, can help meet your needs.

Note: If you are a vegetarian or vegan, the plant source of omega-3, ALA, can also benefit sperm health. Seventy-five grams per day of whole-shelled walnuts (about 18 walnuts) for 12 weeks resulted in improvements in sperm vitality, motility, and morphology.[14]

CoENZYME Q10

CoQ10 stands out with the most robust and compelling data to support its use for improving sperm quality. Sperm motility, morphology, and fertilization rates have all been shown to improve after CoQ10 supplementation. CoQ10 has a specific impact on sperm motility. In one study, participants experienced a 19 percent increase in sperm motility after 6 months of supplementation.[15]

CoQ10 acts as a powerful antioxidant, protecting sperm from damage caused by oxidation. It also plays a crucial role in producing energy within the mitochondria, the powerhouse of cells. This energy production is vital for maintaining the vigorous movement of sperm, known as motility. Without sufficient CoQ10, sperm cells struggle to generate the energy they need for production and movement.

Use and dosage: Between 200 and 600 mg, in soft gel form, taken with a meal containing fat for best absorption.

VITAMIN D

Vitamin D has been shown to benefit sperm health by helping them move better, have the right shape, and improve their ability to fertilize an egg.[16] Low levels of vitamin D have been linked to higher levels of sperm DNA damage, which can affect fertility.[17]

Use and dosage: Taking a vitamin D supplement is all about finding the perfect balance—not too little, not too much, just like Goldilocks. In one study, researchers discovered a "u" shape relationship with sperm and vitamin D. This means that poor sperm parameters were observed *both* at low and at high vitamin D levels. The sweet spot for vitamin D levels appears to be between 32 and 40 ng/mL.[18] The best way to find out where you stand is to get your levels tested!

If your levels are lower, consider taking an additional vitamin D_3 supplement in the range of 1,000–3,000 IUs (25–75 mcg) and retest in 3 months. Don't take more than 4,000 IU (100 mcg) daily without supervision from your doctor, and make sure you account for all supplement sources.

JACK AND EMILY'S STORIES
Creating a Supplement Plan

A personalized supplement plan supports your fertility without crowding your medicine cabinet with every available option. Let's explore the tailored plans for Jack and Emily, each addressing their specific needs and goals.

JACK

Jack's semen analysis showed his sperm count was good, but his sperm motility and morphology were at the low end of normal. Here's how we supported Jack and his swimmers.

No multivitamin needed. Jack was making great progress fueling his fertility with food; he was now eating six to eight servings of veggies per day, with a great balance of protein and healthy fats, so we decided not to add in a multivitamin. He was covered!

Fish oil. A blend of EPA and DHA with a total of 2 g per day to help with motility, morphology, and DNA fragmentation.

CoQ10. 200 mg, two times per day in a soft gel form, taken with a meal. CoQ10 can have a profound effect on sperm motility, something we want to improve for Jack.

Vitamin D. Jack's vitamin D levels were 36 ng/dL (right in the middle of the recommended range for sperm and fertility) so we included a 1,000 mg vitamin D supplement to maintain.

EMILY

The first step of Emily's supplement plan was to get her on a high-quality, pre-natal multivitamin ASAP. The one she was taking before we met was okay (it had 400 mcg of folic acid, so she was reducing the risk of neural tube defects), but it had artificial colors and no choline. Here's how we customized her plan.

Multivitamin. We started her on a new prenatal multivitamin that included 2,000 IU of vitamin D, 300 mg of choline, 27 mg of iron, 400 mcg of folic acid, 400 mcg of methylated folate, and no artificial colors, taken with food. She didn't experience any constipation or nausea from the iron, so no need to supplement separately.

Vitamin D. Emily's vitamin D levels were 42 ng/dL, so we didn't need to add more on top of what was included in the prenatal.

Choline. The two to three eggs per day that Emily eats in addition to the 300 mg in the prenatal vitamin meant she was sure to meet her goal of at least 450 mg of choline daily. No need for an additional choline supplement.

Fish oil. We added a 1 g fish oil capsule that included a combination of DHA and EPA daily, taken with food.

CoQ10. Emily's main concern was egg quality due to her age. She was 34 and CoQ10 levels can start to decline after age 30. We added 200 mg of CoQ10 daily, taken with food.

Probiotic. Emily had a history of taking ibuprofen for menstrual cramps, which can affect the gut microbiome. So in addition to more probiotic-rich foods in her diet, we added a probiotic supplement with 25 billion CFUs and a diversity of strains.

CHAPTER 8

HERBS

FOR EVERYONE

....

Improving Egg and Sperm Health and Beyond

Long before modern medicine existed, plants and herbal remedies were the primary source for health and healing and, in some cultures, still are. Herbs have helped people on their journey, from trying to conceive through postpartum (and beyond) for centuries.

Choosing Herbs That Are Suited to You

Herbs can help affect many aspects of health, including energy, stress, sleep, digestion, endurance, mood, the immune system, and more. Blending centuries of herbal wisdom with the latest scientific research, I try to avoid reductionist thinking of "this herb for this ailment" and instead support the whole person and their individual constitution.

Each herb is unique in its range of benefits, and matching the right herbs for your specific health patterns will result in a more powerful combination. Throughout this chapter, you will learn how several herbs can help support a particular aspect of your fertility. While your immediate goal may be a positive pregnancy test, remember, you are more than just your reproductive parts.

The herbs in this chapter were selected because they are nutritional power-houses, packed with the antioxidants, vitamins, and minerals typically missing from our daily diets. They help support overall health as well as fertility, often by supporting egg and sperm quality. And while our focus is fertility, these are herbs that almost everyone would benefit from incorporating into their life for a myriad of health benefits.

So how do you decide which is best for you . . . or should you just take them all?

No need to mix up a cup of "every herb in this chapter" tea. The goal is to choose the ones that are a good fit for you and your circumstances. For example, some herbs are energizing; that's great, unless you're someone who tends toward feeling overstimulated or has trouble sleeping. In my practice, I look for herbs that will address more than one health concern. If a person who is supporting their fertility also has reflux and constipation, I will choose different herbs for them than for someone who comes in for the same primary concern but gets frequent colds and tends to feel anxious. This is referred to as side benefits as opposed to side effects.

Herbal Energetics

Another consideration when choosing an herb is energetics. Herbal energetics is a way of describing how an herb acts and feels in the body. Herbs can be hot, cold, moist, dry, or neutral. If you have ever eaten a spicy meal with cayenne pepper and felt yourself "heat up," possibly breaking a sweat, you've just experienced an herb with hot energetics. Peppermint is a cooling herb with the opposite effect. When drinking a cup of black tea you may notice your mouth feels a bit dry, while chia seeds feel more moistening. If you tend to feel warm most of the time, warming herbs may feel uncomfortable, but cooling herbs will feel better. Some herbs are energetically neutral, working well for most people's constitutions. Throughout this chapter, the energetics of an herb will be part of the description, when relevant, to help you narrow down the list of herbs to support both your constitution and your fertility.

YOUR RESPONSE MAY VARY

The herbs presented in this book are generally regarded as safe, and most have been used for centuries as both food and medicine. However, individual responses to an herb can vary. Always talk with your doctor or healthcare professional if you are on medications or have a health condition. Not all herbs are considered safe to continue once you are pregnant. Refer to page 104 for herbs that are safe in pregnancy.

Ways to Consume Herbs

You can incorporate herbs into your daily routine in several different ways, and there are pros and cons to each. At the end of the day, the best way to take an herb is whatever way allows you to be consistent. The most common forms that herbs come in are teas, tinctures (alcohol extract), powders, and capsules (powdered whole herb or standardized extract of herbal constituents).

Tea. Teas are a common, inexpensive, and generally accessible way to incorporate herbs into your daily routine. Typical dosage: ½–1 tablespoon of loose-leaf tea per 8 ounces of water, 1–4 cups per day.

Tincture. An herbal tincture is a concentrated liquid form of an herb typically made by steeping the herb in alcohol. Tinctures are a popular and convenient way to take herbs, often providing higher doses than you can get from tea, and are easily digested and absorbed. Herbal tinctures are taken by squirting the desired amount into a few ounces of water and then drinking. The small amount of alcohol present in a tincture typically isn't an issue for most people, but if someone is avoiding alcohol for religious or other reasons, alcohol-free tinctures in glycerine form may be an option. Dosage range will depend on the herb, but it is typically 1–5 mL, two or three times per day. For reference, 1 mL is about 30 drops, and 5 mL is 1 teaspoon. If your tincture bottle has a dropper cap, you can use it to help measure. When you squeeze and release the bulb on the dropper, it will fill with about 1 mL, or 30 drops. You will also hear this referred to as a dropperful.

Powdered herbs. Not all herbs are available in powdered form, but for the ones that are, this is an easy way to incorporate them into your smoothies, hot beverages, baked goods, or glass of water. Dosage range will depend on the herb but is typically 2–10 g per day. Every herb will have a different volume-to-weight ratio, so it is important to follow the dosage guidelines for each individual herb.

Herbal capsules. Capsules come in whole-herb form or as standardized extracts (where only certain herbal constituents are extracted, often in higher dose). The benefit to capsules is convenience. Potential downsides are cost, the volume of capsules you may need to take to get a medicinal dose, and your body's ability to digest and break down capsules. The dosage will vary depending on the herb and if it is in whole form or standardized extract, so follow the dosage on the label.

Green Tea

Green tea (*Camellia sinensis*) is one of the most common teas in the world. Traditionally from China, green tea was once considered a precious medicine only available to the most elite members of society. Today you will find this tea in most grocery stores. It is associated with a host of health benefits, with science supporting what ancient cultures have known for centuries. Green, white, oolong, and black tea are all derived from the same plant species, but they differ in their fermentation and aging processes, which in turn affects the concentration of some beneficial phytonutrients.

High in Phytonutrients

Phytonutrients are plant-based compounds (also known as phytochemicals) that have a beneficial effect on the body. When health experts say "eat the rainbow," they are referring to making sure you get a full spectrum of phytonutrients from different fruits, veggies, and herbs to reap a range of health benefits. Green tea is particularly high in phytonutrients with antioxidant properties, and as you recall from Chapters 2 and 3, antioxidants have a significant impact on egg and sperm quality through their ability to reduce oxidative stress.

Phytonutrients can be broken down into categories based on their chemical structure. Polyphenols are one of those categories. Polyphenols reduce the damage caused by oxidative stress and have a significant effect on improving the body's antioxidant and immune functions.[1] Green tea is so high in polyphenols that 1 cup of tea provides the same amount as about 3 cups of fruit![2]

Polyphenols Support Fertility

Green tea polyphenols possess antioxidant properties that help reduce oxidative stress and improve both egg and sperm quality.[3]

EGCG improves sperm parameters. One of the polyphenols in green tea is called epigallocatechin gallate (EGCG). As an antioxidant, EGCG has been shown to improve sperm parameters in several animal studies.[4] A human in vitro study, where sperm was exposed to EGCG from green tea, demonstrated that EGCG can improve the quality of sperm, particularly sperm motility and viability.[5]

EGCG and egg quality. Supplementation with EGCG has been shown to improve egg quality and embryos, as well as fertilization and pregnancy rates in animal and in vitro studies.[6] This is likely due, at least in part, to EGCG's powerful antioxidant activity.

Although there is more research to be done, it is safe to say the antioxidants in green tea help decrease oxidative stress, which is good for eggs and sperm.

> Other side benefits of green tea: It boosts
> metabolism and burns fat, lowers blood sugar and
> cholesterol levels, fights viral infections, and is
> associated with lower rates of cancer.

EGCG AND LIVER TOXICITY?

EGCG made headlines for studies that have linked it to liver toxicity, but that occurred with very high doses of EGCG extract.[7] Liver toxicity has not been seen in people drinking green tea, even in large quantities. Simply put, this shows how a single component is very different from the synergy of the entire plant.

How to Incorporate Green Tea into Your Routine

Drinking two to three servings of organic green tea per day is a simple and powerful way to support fertility, not to mention your overall health. It is not uncommon for people who start drinking more green tea to boost their fertility to also see the benefits of better energy and staying healthy through cold or flu season (thank you, polyphenols!).

Swapping out some, or all, of your coffee for green tea, with about a third of the caffeine, is smart for your fertility and overall health. One 8-ounce cup of tea averages 20–30 mg of caffeine versus 90–140 mg per 8-ounce cup of coffee.

WILL DECAF WORK?

Does decaffeinated green tea have the same health benefits? If you are sensitive to caffeine, be aware that decaffeinated green tea still has 2–5 mg of caffeine. It is still beneficial for your fertility and overall health, but the benefits depend on the method used to decaffeinate the tea. Chemical decaffeination can strip the tea of up to 70 percent of its antioxidants, significantly decreasing any health benefits. Choosing a certified organic tea is a better option. These are decaffeinated using a carbon dioxide or natural water method and only decrease antioxidant levels by about 5 percent.

Choose the Best Brew for You

If you've tried green tea but not enjoyed the flavor, I encourage you to experiment with different types. Slight variations in where the leaves are grown and how they are processed create unique flavors. Create your own blend, try different loose-leaf varieties, or buy organic tea bags; the benefits are prevalent in whatever form you make your brew. Common types of green tea are sencha, jasmine, green pearl, gunpowder green, dao ren, and matcha.

BREWING TIPS

Green tea should be brewed with *almost*-boiling water (180°F/82°C). Brewing green tea with water that is too hot can increase the amount of tannins in your tea, which can lead you to feel nauseous. If this is a problem for you, make sure you are brewing at the ideal temperature and drink the tea after meals.

Don't steep it for too long, as this can lead to a bitter, unpleasant tasting cup of tea. The ideal time is 3 minutes.

Try adding honey or a squirt of lemon juice to find a flavor you enjoy.

Green Tea Blend

Here is my personal favorite loose-leaf green tea blend. Combining the subtle grassy notes of sencha green tea with the lighter, floral hints of jasmine creates a smooth, just slightly bitter, wonderfully delicious tea!

- 1   cup sencha green tea (mildly bitter, grassy, sharp flavor)
- 1   cup jasmine green tea (distinct floral jasmine flavor)

Mix together and store in a glass jar with a lid.

To prepare a cup of tea, place 1 tablespoon of the tea blend in a mesh tea basket in a mug. Add 8 ounces of almost-boiling water. Cover and steep for 3 minutes. Remove the tea basket and enjoy.

DOES GREEN TEA DECREASE THE ABSORPTION OF FOLATE?

There are some alarmist claims circulating the internet that green tea should be avoided when trying to conceive and in pregnancy because it interferes with the absorption of folate and could increase your baby's risk of a neural tube defect (NTD).

Sounds pretty scary, right? Don't believe everything you read!

Rest assured the available evidence *does not* support this claim. Green tea is the most popular beverage in China and Japan (second to water), and we do not see an increased prevalence of NTDs in those countries.

A systematic review and meta-analysis in 2022 found *no* association between green tea consumption and NTDs.[8] A meta-analysis is a study that combines and analyzes the findings from multiple individual studies, drawing a more robust conclusion and identifying patterns that may not be apparent in individual studies alone.

Another study found that people of child-bearing age who drank green tea in China had higher levels of folate,[9] possibly due to the naturally occurring folate in green tea leaves.

My conclusion: There's no reason to believe green tea, in the recommended amount, is unsafe during preconception, conception, or pregnancy. So continue to take your prenatal multivitamin, separate from other medications, herbs, and some supplements, and enjoy a cup of your favorite green tea.

Matcha Green Tea

Matcha green tea comes from the same tea plant but is processed differently and ground into a powder. With matcha, the ground tea leaves are fully ingested, versus green tea where the leaves are steeped then removed after only a few minutes. This means all of the nutrients, including caffeine, are consumed. Matcha green tea may contain anywhere from 3 to 10 times the quantity of antioxidants contained in standard green tea. It also contains slightly more caffeine than its loose-leaf cousin, but still less than coffee by about 50 percent.

Matcha Latte

1-3 teaspoons matcha powder

2 ounces almost-boiling water

Maple syrup or honey (optional)

½ cup nondairy milk, such as almond or oat, at room temperature or warmed

Place the matcha into a mug (start with 1 teaspoon and work up based on your taste preference). Slowly add the hot water to the matcha powder as you whisk thoroughly. Add the maple syrup (if using) and whisk until dissolved. Gradually whisk in the milk until the latte is smooth and frothy. Serve warm or pour over ice and let chill.

Rooibos

Rooibos (*Aspalathus linearis*) is an indigenous South African plant well known for its use as a naturally caffeine-free herbal tea and increasingly studied for a range of health benefits. Red rooibos (pronounced ROY-boss) gets its color from the fermentation process and is popular for its sweet, nutty, and fruity flavor.

Aspalathin: Polyphenol Superstar

The health benefits of rooibos tea are linked to its high amounts of polyphenol antioxidants, which scavenge free radicals and neutralize reactive oxygen species. Remember the polyphenol antioxidant superstar in green tea called EGCG? Rooibos has its own superstar polyphenol called aspalathin. Interestingly, aspalathin has not been found in any other plant or food source in the world. But, like all herbs, we shouldn't reduce the health benefits of rooibos down to one characteristic. It's likely that all of the antioxidant compounds work together to produce the positive effects associated with this tea.

With regard to the fertility factor, animal and in vitro studies of rooibos have shown improvements in sperm concentration and motility,[10] ovarian functions,[11] and protection from negative effects of exposure during pregnancy to bisphenol A (BPA),[12] a toxin found in plastics (more on environmental exposures in Chapter 10).

Side benefits include blood sugar balance and reduced insulin resistance, beneficial effects on blood pressure, and reduction of inflammation. The potent antioxidant content in rooibos tea may even help protect against the free radical damage associated with cancer.

A Brew for All

Revered for its antioxidant properties, rooibos is a healthy tea for everyone. With health benefits similar to green tea, rooibos is a tasty, caffeine-free alternative for people who don't like the slightly bitter flavor of green tea.

Rooibos tea should be steeped for at least 10 minutes for full flavor and health benefits. Enjoy 2–4 cups of rooibos tea daily.

Cacao-Rooibos Tea

The flavor of rooibos tea is delicious on its own but also pairs well with chocolate and vanilla. This recipe adds cacao nibs and a dash of vanilla extract to red rooibos for a delicious tea that also satisfies a sweet tooth. Cacao is also high in antioxidants, and some studies have shown it can decrease oxidative stress. All good for the soul, the body, and fertility!

- 1 tablespoon red rooibos tea
- 1 teaspoon cacao nibs
- 8 ounces boiling water
  Dash of pure vanilla extract

Combine the tea and cacao in a mesh tea basket in a mug. Add the boiling water and vanilla. Cover and steep for 10-15 minutes. Remove the tea basket and enjoy.

Oat Straw

You might be familiar with oats as a hot breakfast option, but the oat plant (*Avena sativa*) offers so much more! Herbalists work with both the immature oat seed, known as milky oat tops, and the dried oat stalk, referred to as oat straw. They both support the nervous system and have a long list of unique benefits, but the dried oat straw stands out for its nutrient-dense and nourishing support. Rich in antioxidants and minerals such as silica, calcium, magnesium, and iron, as well as B vitamins and folic acid, oat straw is like a multivitamin in the form of a tea.

Energetically, oat straw is neutral (not too warm, not too cool) and moistening. Its mild hay flavor is slightly sweet and tastes lovely on its own but also blends well with other more drying herbs for balance.

Oat straw offers other benefits, as well. It lowers stress, reduces premenstrual cramps, helps balance blood sugar and decrease sugar cravings, and strengthens hair, nails, teeth, and bones.

WHEN TO AVOID OAT STRAW

Oat straw is extremely safe, unless you are allergic to oats—in which case, it should be avoided. Also, if you have a gluten sensitivity, approach with caution. While oats don't include gluten, they do contain a protein that is similar to proteins found in wheat. Oat crops can also be cross-contaminated with gluten from nearby farms or processing facilities.

Oat Straw Infusion

Sipping on an oat straw infusion is calming and nourishing, but you will get the best results if you drink oats daily, over several months. I like to make my infusion in the evening. It steeps overnight and can be enjoyed throughout the following day.

1 cup dried oat straw
3-4 cardamom pods (optional, for flavor)
32 ounces (4 cups) boiling water

Place the oat straw and cardamom pods (if using) in a 32-ounce glass jar with a lid or in a large French press. Fill with the boiling water. Put the lid on and let steep for at least 4 hours or overnight. Use a mesh strainer or the French press to strain out the herbs. Drink at the temperature you prefer (room temperature, warm, or cold over ice). Store leftover infusion in the refrigerator and drink within 24 hours.

Nettle

Nettle (*Urtica dioica*) leaf, also called stinging nettles, is known for the sting encountered when you brush up against this common "weed." This plant is revered by herbalists for all of its nutritive and medicinal gifts. Nettle is a nutrient-dense herb, rich in easily absorbable vitamins A, C, E, and K, and notably the minerals calcium, magnesium, silica, iron, and zinc. Nettle provides nutrients likely missing from our diet and required for optimal fertility. A strong nettle infusion is a great way to "drink your greens" and up your fertility game at the same time.

Nettle offers other side benefits as well. It supports blood sugar balance, relieves seasonal allergies, and improves energy.

Many of my clients are surprised to discover how much they enjoy working with nettle to support their fertility, and they find it's something they stick with for years, as nettles are an herbal ally through many of life's stages, including:

- Preconception: antioxidants for egg and sperm health

- Pregnancy: nutrient-dense qualities to support healthy energy levels, increased nutritional demands, and iron levels

- Postpartum: builds back energy

- Lactation: increases milk flow and nourishment for the nursing parent and baby

- Perimenopause and menopause: high concentrations of bioabsorbable calcium and magnesium for bone health

Energetically, nettle is cooling and quite drying. It can be too drying on its own for some people, but combining it with moistening and neutral herbs can help balance this effect. See the recipe for an overnight infusion of nettle and oat straw (a nutrient-dense herb in its own right, also high in antioxidants, vitamins, and minerals) on page 92.

Simple Overnight Nettle Infusion

This highly potent tea is made by steeping a generous amount of nettle herb for several hours or overnight. The result is a strong, medicinal drink that packs a powerful nutritive punch.

- ¾   cup dried nettle leaf
- 32   ounces (4 cups) boiling water

Place the nettle in a 32-ounce glass jar with a lid or in a large French press. Fill with the boiling water. Put the lid on and let steep for at least 4 hours or overnight. Use a mesh strainer or the French press to strain out the herbs. Drink at the temperature you prefer (room temperature, warm, or cold over ice). Store leftover infusion in the refrigerator and drink within 24 hours.

Nettle Matcha Latte

This version of a matcha latte is an antioxidant-packed green drink. Adding powdered nettle to the latte means that you consume all of the herbs, as opposed to a tea or infusion where the leaves are steeped and removed. It also means the drink can be a bit thick or "grainy" with some green goodness left at the bottom of your glass. The more you mix, the less residue you will end up with. You can make this drink in a blender or with a whisk, and drink it hot or over ice.

- 1–3   teaspoons matcha powder
- ¼   cup dried nettle leaf, ground to a powder with spice grinder or blender (or 1½ tablespoons powdered nettle)
- ½   cup almost-boiling water
    Maple syrup or honey (optional)
- ½   cup nondairy milk, such as almond or oat (warmed, if desired)

Place the matcha (start with 1 teaspoon and work up based on taste preference) and nettle in a mug. Slowly add the hot water to the powder as you whisk thoroughly. Add the maple syrup, if using, and whisk until dissolved. Gradually mix in the milk and whisk until the latte is smooth and frothy. Serve warm or pour over ice.

Alternatively, prepare the latte in a blender: Combine the matcha and nettle in a blender and pulse to combine. Add the hot water and blend well. Add the maple syrup to taste, if using, and the milk, and blend a final time.

Overnight Nettle and Oat Straw Infusion

A beautiful balance between nettle's drying and oat straw's moistening energetics, this overnight infusion is a nutritive blend full of antioxidants, vitamins, and minerals. The addition of peppermint helps shift the flavor from earthy and grassy to a bit minty.

- ½ cup dried oat straw
- ¼ cup dried nettle leaf
- 1 tablespoon dried spearmint or peppermint leaf (optional, for flavor)
- 32 ounces (4 cups) boiling water

Combine the herbs in a 32-ounce glass jar with a lid or in a French press. Fill with the boiling water. Put the lid on and let steep for at least 4 hours or overnight. Use a mesh strainer or the French press to strain out the herbs. Drink 2 cups per day at the temperature you prefer (warm, room temperature, or cold over ice). Store leftover infusion in the refrigerator and drink within 24 hours.

Variation: Want to save time? Make a large batch of this herbal mixture at once. Purchase 8 ounces or up to 1 pound each of the dried herbs, then mix in a ratio of 1 part dried oat straw to ½ part dried nettle leaf. Mix all the herbs together and store in an airtight container in a cool, dark place. Scoop out about ¾ cup of the mixture when making your overnight infusion.

Turmeric

Turmeric (*Curcuma longa*) is famous for its vibrant yellow color and use as a spice in curries and other Indian, Middle Eastern, and Southeast Asian cuisine. In addition to its culinary uses, turmeric has been used for medicinal purposes for centuries.

Turmeric's potential health benefits caught the attention of medical researchers in the late twentieth century, and since then, thousands of studies have been conducted. Turmeric, with its notorious phytonutrient curcumin, is by far one of the most studied medicinal herbs. Curcumin gets a lot of press for its powerful anti-inflammatory and antioxidant activity. It has been shown to have potential benefits for a range of health conditions, including cancer, Alzheimer's disease, arthritis, inflammation, digestive disorders, anxiety, and depression.

A Powerful Antioxidant

As a potent antioxidant, curcumin helps undo the damage of free radicals and decrease oxidative stress. Remember, oxidative stress is the enemy of healthy egg and sperm development. A clinical trial showed curcumin significantly increased total sperm count and motility levels, along with supporting a remarkable improvement in overall antioxidant activity.[13] There are also several in vitro studies showing that curcumin improves sperm motility,[14,15] likely through its protection against oxidative stress.

Both sperm and eggs, while seemingly distinct, are fundamentally the same type of cell (called a gamete). So while there's not a lot of research on turmeric and egg quality, it's reasonable to assume that what is good for the sperm is good for the egg.

With such a long list of overall health benefits, it's not hard to find reasons to add turmeric to your daily routine. Several studies have confirmed curcumin can reduce muscle soreness and inflammation after exercise.[16] In my practice, I have seen it work as well as, if not better than, ibuprofen for exercise-related achiness, without the risk of stomach upset or disruption of healthy gut bacteria that can occur from regular use of pain relievers.

After reading this section, you may be thinking, "Turmeric lattes for everyone!" As a general rule, most people would benefit from adding ½ teaspoon of this herb into their cooking or drinking "golden milk" (see the recipe, page 94) each day, but to get the medicinal doses shown to be effective in studies, you will need to take a capsule of either turmeric powder or curcumin extract.

Warning: Turmeric may have antiplatelet and blood-thinning effect, so avoid medicinal doses of turmeric if you are taking blood thinners or have a blood-clotting disorder, and discontinue medicinal use at least 2 weeks prior to undergoing surgery. Use caution if you have a history of gallstones or bile duct obstruction.

What's the Best Form: Turmeric or Curcumin Extract?

While many studies (and supplement companies) focus solely on curcumin, a growing number of studies have shown curcumin is not the only medicinally active or beneficial component in turmeric. In fact, taking an isolated curcumin supplement could mean you are missing out on many of the other well-documented benefits of turmeric. Consuming turmeric in its whole form provides nearly 300 other beneficial components. Look for brands listing the root or root extract (often listed as *Curcuma longa* root extract) standardized for 95 percent curcuminoids. Black pepper (*Piper nigrum*) is helpful for the optimal absorption of turmeric, so choose a supplement that also includes black pepper.

Typical Dosage Ranges

Powder: 2–10 g (1 teaspoon equals about 3.5 g) per day

Tincture: 4–6 mL, two or three times per day

Capsules: Follow the recommended dosage on the label; 250–500 mg capsule, two or three times per day

CURCUMIN AND ITS EFFECT ON SPERM

If you start searching online for "fertility and turmeric" you may find yourself down a rabbit hole of studies and headlines claiming turmeric or curcumin is harmful to sperm. Some researchers have even suggested that turmeric could be used as a spermicide or contraceptive! If you read the fine print, the antifertility effects were dose dependent and reversible after stopping treatment.

A few animal studies have shown that high doses of curcumin have a negative effect on spermatogenesis and sperm parameters. However, these studies involved administering very high doses of curcumin, which are not typically consumed through dietary sources or supplementation.

Most studies were in vitro studies (curcumin exposed to sperm in a petri dish).[17,18] The dose required to achieve a toxic effect on sperm cells was described as "unattainable in the organism," meaning the dose was so high that it cannot be reached within the body. Other studies fed mice a turmeric extract and found antifertility effects at doses between 500 and 600 mg per kg of weight.[19,20] To put this into perspective, the equivalent dose for a 150-pound person would be 34–40 g, or 3½–4 tablespoons.

Golden Milk

Golden milk is a traditional Ayurvedic beverage combining milk, turmeric, and spices. This is my favorite recipe, but you could purchase premade, organic golden milk blends that are delicious, too.

- 1 cup nondairy milk
- 1 teaspoon coconut oil or ghee
- ½ teaspoon ground turmeric
- ¼ teaspoon ground ginger
- ¼ teaspoon ground cinnamon
- ¼ teaspoon ground cardamom
- ¼ teaspoon ground nutmeg
- 1-2 twists of freshly ground black pepper
- Honey (optional)

Heat the milk, oil, and spices in a saucepan until hot but not boiling. Add honey to taste. Mix (by hand or in a blender) to combine well and make frothy. Drink hot.

Ashwagandha

Ashwagandha (*Withania somnifera*) has been used for thousands of years in Ayurvedic medicine, an ancient system of healing that originated in India. Ashwagandha is known for its adaptogenic properties, which means it helps the body adapt to stress and restore balance. Today ashwagandha root is used around the world to manage anxiety, stress, inflammation, low libido, and infertility, and support sleep, immune function, and overall vitality.

With its long history of use as an aphrodisiac and fertility enhancer, researchers wanted to know if this herb was worthy of the hype, and if so, how it worked. What they found circles back to oxidative stress and hormones.

Decreases Oxidative Stress

Ashwagandha was found to fight the formation of reactive oxygen species and increase antioxidant levels, leading to a decrease in oxidative stress.[21] As you know from Chapters 2 and 3, oxidative stress is bad for eggs and sperm. Healthy levels of testosterone are also important for sperm production (and a healthy libido), and ashwagandha helps increase testosterone levels.[22] Fun fact: Ashwagandha improves testosterone levels in people who are low in this hormone, but not in people with normal levels for whom an increase could be unhealthy. How cool is that?

Increases Semen Volume and Improves Sleep

Clinical studies found ashwagandha significantly increased semen volume, sperm count (by a whopping 167 percent!), and motility (improved by 57 percent)[23,24] and improved libido[25] after only 3 months of consistent use.

A discussion about ashwagandha wouldn't be complete without talking about its superpower to help people get a better night's sleep. Ashwagandha's Latin species name, *somnifera*, means "sleep-inducing." When taken consistently over time, this herb can help promote a better quality of sleep. We will talk more about sleep and its impact on fertility in Chapter 9.

With a robust list of side benefits, ashwagandha is an herb that makes its way into many of my clients' holistic herbal plans. It is a wonderful herbal ally for people who are not only looking to start a family but are tired, anxious, frazzled, or stressed out.

How to Take It

In the Ayurvedic tradition, ashwagandha is most commonly taken as a powder mixed into milk or other foods, but it can also be taken as a supplement or in tincture form. Add it to smoothies, the Golden Milk recipe (see page 94), or swap out maca for ashwagandha in the Maca Nut Butter Balls recipe (see page 99).

Warning: Ashwagandha is part of the nightshade family, so if you react negatively to nightshade plants, you may want to avoid it or start with very small doses to see how you feel. Examples of foods in the nightshade family include tomatoes, white potatoes, all peppers (except black pepper), eggplant, goji berries, paprika, and chili powder. In my experience, most people with nightshade sensitivities can tolerate ashwagandha without issue.

Typical Dosage Ranges

Powder: 2–6 g (1 teaspoon equals about 2.5 g) per day

Tincture: 4–6 mL, two or three times per day

Capsules: 250–500 mg, two to four times per day

Chocolate Banana Almond Smoothie

Cinnamon and chocolate pair beautifully with the slightly bitter flavor of ashwagandha, while the banana adds just the right amount of sweetness. This smoothie is one of my favorites for the colder months since it isn't as icy as other smoothies. Feel free to add a handful of ice if you prefer it colder.

½ banana
1 cup almond milk, plus more if needed
¼ cup almond butter
2 tablespoons cacao powder
1 teaspoon ashwagandha powder
1 teaspoon ground cinnamon
1 teaspoon pure vanilla extract

Place all the ingredients in a blender. Blend, adding more almond milk if needed for your desired consistency.

Maca

Not to be confused with matcha, maca (*Lepidium meyenii*) is a plant native to the Andean mountains of Peru. The root has been used by Indigenous peoples as a source of food and medicine for years. Incan warriors used to consume maca before battle, and Peruvian children are fed maca porridge to support brain growth and build muscle. It is a nutritive herb that has a long history of use to increase energy, libido, sexual function, and fertility.

A Wildly Popular Superfood

Until recently, maca was relatively unknown outside of its native area. Its popularity skyrocketed in the 1990s when it was marketed to improve sexual function and overall vitality. This has led to local harvesting issues, price increases, and in some cases, overhyped marketing claims of the next superfood.

Maca's notoriety for its potential to enhance libido and sexual function has led to its reputation as a "natural Viagra" for the treatment of erectile dysfunction. Although studies support maca's effect on libido[26,27] and erectile dysfunction,[28] exactly how it works isn't clear. One small study showed an increase in seminal volume, sperm count, and sperm motility after 4 months.[29] A larger trial found a 15–20 percent increase in sperm parameters after 3 months.[30] The studies on maca and fertility are limited but encouraging.

Source Maca Carefully

Maca has been consumed safely in traditional South American cultures in quite high dosages (20–100 g per day) without reported negative side effects. However, since the explosion of maca's popularity, concerns regarding sourcing and quality are on the rise. To ensure that you are ingesting a safe and effective product, choose organic maca from a reputable source that has a direct relationship with Peruvian farmers. Some companies source maca from China, which may not be as effective or safe.

Maca is a highly nutritious herb with a long safety record. It is rich in essential amino acids, potassium, calcium, magnesium, iron, and zinc—all important building blocks for optimal egg and sperm production. Adding maca powder to your morning smoothie, coffee, or other foods is an easy way to boost many of these essential nutrients.

Typical Dosage Ranges

Powder: 2–8 g (1 teaspoon equals about 4 g) per day
Tincture: 4–6 mL, two or three times per day
Capsules: 250–500 mg, two to four times per day

MACA OPTIONS

When considering maca options, it's helpful to understand the differences between raw and gelatinized forms, as well as the potential significance of the various maca root colors.

What's the Difference between Raw and Gelatinized Maca?

Traditionally, maca roots are dried in the sun after harvesting and then boiled or cooked before being eaten. Raw maca powder is produced by drying the roots naturally or with a low-temperature dehydrator, then grinding them into a fine powder. Raw maca is never heated above 105°F (41°C), thereby preserving the maximum amount of nutrients. However, raw maca contains starch, which can sometimes be difficult to digest.

Gelatinized maca is a newer method of preparation where the roots are boiled first, then pressurized to remove all starch content, making the powder easier to digest. The lack of starch means that gram for gram, gelatinized maca is more concentrated than raw maca powders, so the nutrient density is higher. But high heat destroys all enzymes, vitamin C content, and glucosinolates (compounds that help protect your cells from free radical damage).

When it comes to choosing, both raw and gelatinized maca powders have been used in studies with equally mixed results. In my experience, both work well; however, if you have trouble digesting raw maca, choose gelatinized maca powder. It's more important to choose a high-quality, organic brand than to worry about raw versus gelatinized.

Does the Color of the Maca Matter?

Maca root can have a variety of colors, and the color of the root may influence its health properties. Yellow maca is the most common and most widely used. Red and black maca are other colors you may find. There isn't enough research to clearly establish one color as "better" than another for egg or sperm health and fertility.

Maca Nut Butter Balls

Nut butter balls are a delicious and convenient way to incorporate powdered herbs into a healthy snack option. This recipe makes approximately 40 teaspoon-size balls. Each ball contains roughly 2 grams of maca.

- 1 cup nut butter (almond, cashew, or sunflower)
- ½ cup chopped almonds, plus extra to roll each ball in, if desired
- ½ cup chopped cacao nibs
- ½ cup honey
- ½ cup powdered maca
- ⅓ cup tahini
- 1 tablespoon cacao powder
- 1 teaspoon ground cardamom
- 1 teaspoon ground ginger

In a large bowl, mix together all the ingredients until a thick paste forms. Roll into balls about 1-inch in diameter. Coat with the chopped almonds for extra crunch, if using. Store in the refrigerator, or freeze to eat throughout the month. Eat one to four balls per day.

Variation: This recipe can be modified to include ashwagandha as well. Either combine ¼ cup maca and ¼ cup ashwagandha, or swap out the maca entirely for ashwagandha.

Astragalus

Astragalus (*Astragalus mongholicus*) root has been used in traditional Chinese medicine (TCM) to enhance the body's natural immune system and promote overall health and vitality. Modern research validates its immune-supportive properties and other health benefits, such as reducing inflammation, improving heart function, protecting against certain types of cancer, and recovering from chemotherapy.[31,32]

Support for Swimmers

From a fertility standpoint, astragalus helps your swimmers swim better. Preliminary in vitro studies demonstrated this herb improves sperm motility[33,34] and an animal study suggests it may work through the regulation of gene expression during spermatogenesis.[35] Astragalus also helps sperm through its high concentration of antioxidants (and their ability to fight oxidative stress), vitamins, and minerals such as folate, choline, iron, magnesium, silicon, and zinc.

Astragalus is one of my top choices for people who are prone to frequent colds, viruses, respiratory infections, or asthma or are recovering from chemotherapy. Admittedly, astragalus is not the first herb I reach for to improve sperm, but if you are trying to support sperm health *and* you could use an immune boost, then consider adding astragalus to the mix.

In TCM, astragalus is a food-based herb taken in relatively large doses over an extended period of time. Many people I work with prefer taking the capsule form for convenience, but a strong cup of tea is a great way to get additional astragalus into your daily diet.

Typical Dosage Ranges

Dried root: 10–30 g of sliced, cut and sifted, or powdered root per day
Tincture: 4–6 mL, two or three times per day
Capsules: 500–1,000 mg, two or three times per day

Astragalus Chai Tea

I find the sweet, woody taste of astragalus blends well with the robust, spicy flavor of chai tea, and I enjoy making mine from scratch and simmering it on the stove to really pull out the flavors and medicinal properties of the astragalus (herbalists call this method a decoction). Side benefit: Your house will smell amazing! You can also steep the herbs in a mug and strain it like other loose-leaf teas. Just be sure to steep your tea for at least 30 minutes in order to get the medicinal benefits, and the longer you steep, the better.

1 teaspoon rooibos tea
½ teaspoon ground ginger
¼ teaspoon ground cinnamon
2 whole cloves
2 cardamom pods
1 whole star anise

10-20 g sliced astragalus (20-30 slices)
Pinch of nutmeg
Honey or maple syrup (optional)

Pour 2 cups of water and all of the herbs into a saucepan. Bring to a boil, reduce heat to a simmer, cover, and simmer for 20 minutes. Strain. Sweeten with honey or maple syrup to taste, if desired.

Variation: Looking for a quick tea hack? If the above instructions made you roll your eyes and say, "I'm not fitting this into my crazy day," try this. Add boiling water and a handful of astragalus root slices to a thermos, drop in a chai tea bag, and let steep for 30 minutes before drinking. You can remove the tea bag and leave the astragalus slices in the thermos while you sip on your tea throughout the day.

Ginger

Ginger (*Zingiber officinale*) root is one of the oldest and most revered herbs in the Ayurvedic and TCM traditions and remains one of the most popular herbs of our time. It adds a spicy, aromatic flavor to your cooking and offers numerous health benefits.

Extensive studies have confirmed ginger's efficacy in supporting a wide range of health conditions. It's used for reducing inflammatory pain and menstrual cramps; improving digestion; relieving nausea, migraines, and seasonal allergies; and fighting viral infections. Ginger is also useful for increasing circulation. I find this particularly helpful for clients who spend a lot of time sitting. It helps increase blood flow to the pelvic area and uterus.

Potential for Supporting Sperm

The research on ginger used to support fertility is relatively limited, but there are two clinical studies on sperm health that are encouraging. In one study, the rate of DNA fragmentation was significantly lower after 3 months of treatment.[36] In another study, the use of ginger caused a significant increase in sperm parameters, most notably a 47 percent increase in sperm motility, as well as improvements in fragmentation and hormone levels, including testosterone.[37]

Ginger is loaded with antioxidants and can easily be incorporated into your daily routine. A simple cup of lemon ginger tea contains 1–3 g of ginger. Consider adding ginger to your routine if you sit a lot (in addition to taking more breaks to get up and move around!), feel bloated or gassy after meals, have painful periods, suffer from seasonal allergies, or tend toward feeling cold.

Typical Dosage Ranges

Powder: 3–12 g (1 teaspoon dried powder equals about 2 g) per day
Fresh root: 3–12 g (1 teaspoon fresh root grated or finely chopped equals about 4 g) per day
Tincture: 1–2 mL, two or three times per day
Capsules: 250–500 mg, two to four times per day
Note: Pregnant people should not ingest more than 2 g of ginger per day.

GINGER ISN'T FOR EVERYONE

If you have ever tried a strong ginger tea or enjoyed a meal heavily seasoned with ginger, you may have noticed you felt warmer, perhaps even breaking a sweat. This is a classic example of herbal energetics. Ginger is a warm-to-hot herb that is also drying. If you tend to run warm (in herbalism this is called having a warm constitution), you may find ginger irritating and too heating. Ginger is ideal for people with colder constitutions.

Pregnant people should also use ginger with caution. Ginger may be stimulating to the uterus and could increase the chance of uterine contractions. Although culinary doses of ginger are considered safe for most people, pregnant people should limit their intake to 2 g per day.

Lemon Ginger Tea

This warming, spicy tea is supportive for your sperm and overall health and may turn out to be one of your favorite teas for its versatile health benefits. It is one of the first remedies we reach for in our home if someone has an upset stomach or at the first signs of a sore throat or cold.

1-2 teaspoons grated or chopped fresh ginger (no need to peel)
8 ounces boiling water
   Juice from ½ lemon
   Honey

Place the ginger in a mesh tea basket in a mug. Add the boiling water. Cover and steep for 10-15 minutes. Remove the tea basket and add the lemon juice and honey to taste. Enjoy! Alternatively, if slicing your ginger, you could skip the mesh strainer and let the ginger sink to the bottom of the mug; no need to strain.

Antioxidants are your egg and sperm's
best friends, and herbs are loaded
with antioxidants.

Use the Power of Herbs to Spice It Up

Sometimes you don't have to look farther than the fresh produce aisle or your spice cabinet for powerful remedies to support your fertility. Simply adding more culinary herbs and spices to your diet can have a big impact! As I've discussed throughout this chapter, herbs are high in antioxidants, which help balance oxidative stress and protect and support egg and sperm health.

You really can't go wrong when adding more herbs and spices to your meals. Small amounts can add up over time and have a big impact. In general, you can add a handful of fresh herbs to almost any meal or snack. Experiment with different herbs to see what flavor combinations you enjoy.

Here are a few ideas on how you can spice things up and boost your intake of antioxidants:

- Sprinkle a generous handful of fresh herbs over eggs (basil, thyme, and parsley are delicious) and serve over a bed of arugula.

- Add fresh oregano or thyme to toast with avocado and tomato slices.

- Sprinkle generous handfuls of fresh herbs over your pasta.

- Experiment with fresh herbs in your salad (parsley, oregano, cilantro, thyme, mint, and lemon balm are all wonderful options).

- Serve your protein (chicken, fish, meat) on a bed of greens, such as arugula, parsley, thyme, rosemary, and oregano.

- Add pesto to your protein or pasta (use pesto made from basil, or make your own using parsley, lemon balm, rosemary, or thyme).

- Add cinnamon to your oatmeal or chia pudding.

- Add cinnamon or turmeric to your latte or smoothie.

- When recipes call for fresh ginger or garlic, try doubling the amount.

- Add turmeric to Bolognese or tomato sauce and finish with a handful of fresh basil or parsley.

- Add a handful of mint or lemon balm to a pitcher of water and drink throughout the day.

- Add a sprig of fresh rosemary to hot water with lemon.

Herbal Safety and Pregnancy

All of the herbs presented in this book are safe while trying to conceive, but not all are safe during pregnancy. If you think you are pregnant or you have a positive pregnancy test, refer to the list on the opposite page and stop taking any herbs that are not on this list. The exception to this is culinary doses of herbs and spices in your food, which are perfectly safe. Also note that not all herbs listed are safe with prescription medications. Always check with a qualified practitioner.

HERBAL AUDIT: ENSURING YOUR DAILY ROUTINE IS PREGNANCY-SAFE

Take a close look at everything you consume throughout the day—powders, juices, supplements, teas, protein shakes, and natural energy drinks—to ensure they're free from herbs that may not be safe during pregnancy. For example, fresh juices may contain high amounts of ginger, which is unsafe in large doses during pregnancy. Protein powders or energy blends might include adaptogenic herbs or mushroom extracts that aren't pregnancy-safe. Carefully read ingredient labels and double-check all herbs against the list above. When in doubt, consult a health-care professional with expertise in herbal medicine.

Herbs That Are Safe During Pregnancy

(See exceptions noted on the opposite page.)

- Alfalfa
  (*Medicago sativa*)

- Astragalus
  (*Astragalus mongholicus*)

- Black haw
  (*Viburnum prunifolium*)

- California poppy
  (*Eschscholzia californica*)

- Chamomile
  (*Matricaria chamomilla*)

- Cramp bark
  (*Viburnum opulus*)

- Dandelion root and leaf
  (*Taraxacum officinale*)

- Echinacea
  (*Echinacea angustifolia*)

- Eleuthero
  (*Eleutherococcus senticosus*)

- Ginger
  (*Zingiber officinale*)
  *limit 2 g per day

- Hawthorn
  (*Crataegus* spp.)

- Lavender
  (*Lavandula* spp.)

- Lemon balm
  (*Melissa officinalis*)

- Marshmallow root or leaf
  (*Althaea officinalis*)

- Nettle leaf
  (*Urtica dioica*)

- Oat
  (*Avena sativa*)

- Passionflower
  (*Passiflora incarnata*)

- Peppermint
  (*Mentha × piperita*)

- Plantain
  (*Plantago* spp.)

- Raspberry leaf
  (*Rubus idaeus*) *in the second
  and third trimesters only

- Reishi
  (*Ganoderma lucidum*)

- Shatavari
  (*Asparagus racemosus*)

- Skullcap
  (*Scutellaria lateriflora*)

- Spearmint
  (*Mentha spicata*)

- St. John's wort
  (*Hypericum perforatum*)

- Valerian
  (*Valeriana officinalis*)

- Wild yam
  (*Dioscorea villosa*)

- Yellow dock
  (*Rumex crispus*)

JACK AND EMILY'S STORIES
Herbs to Support Overall Well-Being

Choosing the right herbs goes beyond just addressing specific issues; it's about finding the ones that align with your unique health patterns and constitution, helping you narrow down your list of "every amazing herb" to the herbs that holistically support your overall well-being. Here's how this came together for Jack and Emily.

JACK

When Jack started his herbal protocol, his biggest concern was improving the two sperm parameters that were at the very low end of normal for him: motility and morphology. Through our discussion, I learned that Jack had a stressful job that was taking a toll on his overall health and wellness. He was feeling anxious throughout the day, had trouble falling asleep, often woke up around 3 a.m., and had difficulty getting back to sleep. Jack's fertility plan took all of these things into consideration.

Green tea. Jack was relying on coffee to get himself started in the morning and drinking 2–3 cups throughout the day, with his last cup around 3 p.m. Caffeine can contribute to anxiety, provides zero sustainable energy, and can disrupt sleep in the evening. Jack agreed to cut back to 1 cup of coffee first thing in the morning, and then have 2–3 cups of green tea throughout the day.

Ashwagandha. This herb was a great fit for Jack because its antioxidant properties helped support sperm quality, and as an adaptogen it helped improve his reaction to stress while lowering stress hormones like cortisol (which can contribute to weight gain), decreased his anxiety, and, over time, helped improve his sleep quality. Jack took 1,000 mg of ashwagandha in capsule form every morning.

Maca. As a nutritive herb, this is a great addition to almost anyone's diet, especially since studies have shown improvements in sperm parameters over time. Remember the grab-and-go snacks that Jack discovered in Chapter 6 contained industrial seed oils and trans fats? Maca Nut Butter Balls are a great replacement! To help keep Jack's protocol manageable, Jack and his partner decided to make a large batch of Maca Nut Butter Balls, freeze them, and snack on two to four per day.

Spice it up. Jack committed to adding more greens and spices to the meals he was already eating in order to boost his overall antioxidant and phytonutrient intake.

At our 4-week follow-up, the biggest change Jack noticed was his sleep. He was falling asleep easier and sleeping through most nights. His stress levels at work felt lower, and he was feeling less anxious overall.

EMILY

Emily's main concern was her egg quality. During our initial appointment, she mentioned that the first day of her period could be pretty painful; she often needed to take ibuprofen to get through the day. She also spent a lot of time sitting at the computer and wasn't getting as much exercise as she would like. Here's how we structured Emily's herbal plan:

Nettle. Emily began with the Overnight Nettle and Oat Straw Infusion, which is loaded with antioxidants to support egg quality and general health. At night she made a batch, and she drank 16 ounces at room temperature throughout the next morning.

Ginger. When Emily mentioned painful periods, I immediately thought of ginger. Ginger can help improve blood flow and circulation to the pelvic area. Emily made a cup of the Lemon Ginger Tea every afternoon after lunch. At the first sign of menstrual cramps, she doubled the recipe and drank 2 cups throughout the day. She also purchased ginger capsules and took 1,000 mg two or three times per day on the first day of her period.

Spice it up. I encouraged Emily to use more herbs and spices in her cooking as an easy yet powerful way to boost nutrition, antioxidants, and phytochemicals.

Alarm clock. Emily's job required a lot of seated desk time, so I recommended setting a timer as a reminder to get up and move. This helps increase blood flow to the pelvic area, delivering hormones, nutrients, and oxygen to the ovaries and uterus. Interestingly, ovarian blood flow declines with age, and decreased ovarian blood flow is associated with poorer IVF outcomes.

At our 6-week follow-up, Emily couldn't wait to share that when her period started she had had only mild cramping—not enough to reach for pain medication. If it got bad enough, she took a few ginger capsules and felt better. She was really enjoying the nettle and oat infusion, and noticed an improvement in her overall energy. At our 12-week follow-up, the period pain was a distant memory, and Emily didn't even need the extra ginger capsules after a few months of drinking ginger tea regularly.

CHAPTER 9

STRESS, SLEEP, MOVEMENT, AND MINDFULNESS

Building a Strong Foundation for Fertility

Deciding you're ready to have a baby but not getting pregnant when you thought you would is one of life's biggest stressors. Making a few holistic lifestyle changes—stress management, sufficient sleep, regular movement, and some form of mindfulness—will support your fertility and mental health while you navigate the road to parenthood. Even more importantly, these strategies are good for you as a human.

Stress Is Real

How many times have you heard "Just relax and you'll get pregnant!" (cringe)? Managing stress while trying to conceive is important, but not for the reasons you may think. While there are ways stress affects fertility, the studies are not conclusive regarding the overall impact. One of the perhaps not so obvious ways it can affect your chances of getting pregnant is that stress is one of the most common reasons for the discontinuation of fertility treatments,[1] as people trying to conceive can feel alone and overwhelmed. Stress can also be a contributing factor (although not likely the cause) for certain conditions that affect fertility.

One thing I want you to understand is that stress is more than just an uncomfortable feeling or something you need to push through or manage to get pregnant. Actual physiological and psychological changes occur in the body when we experience stress. Taking it a step further, ongoing stress can affect overall health, wellness, mood, and relationships. Trying to get pregnant can be incredibly stressful, especially if you're experiencing infertility. One study even showed anxiety levels associated with infertility were higher than those for people diagnosed with cancer or heart disease.[2] So it's obvious that stress management during this time is critical.

The bottom line is that it's not just "all in your head." If nothing else, hear this—you don't need to be a martyr. You deserve to feel well in all areas of your life!

The strategies in this chapter are not meant to "hack your stress" in order for you to get pregnant faster; instead they present holistic ways of supporting your body's response to stress. These strategies will help you navigate your journey with more resilience and an overall better quality of life. While you can't control everything, you can have strategies in place to manage stress and help you work through anxiety, depression, and self-esteem issues.

The Stress Response and the Hormone Cascade

Stress is a natural part of life, and the stress response is the body's way of protecting you. The human nervous system has evolved to trigger the "fight, flight, or freeze" response to save us from life-threatening situations. When your bodily response is working properly, stress helps you stay focused, energetic, and alert. In emergency situations, stress can save your life—giving you extra strength to defend yourself or fast reflexes to swerve away from danger.

The same mechanism is activated in the face of an imminent physical danger (i.e., you are terrified of needles and you brace yourself as the phlebotomist draws your fertility lab work) or as a result of a psychological threat (i.e., you are not yet pregnant and are on the drive to another baby shower) or a perceived threat (i.e., it's taking longer than you thought to get pregnant and you fear it'll never happen).

The Science Behind the Stress Response

The body's response to stress starts in the brain. This is the beginning of a feedback loop that occurs along the hypothalamic-pituitary-adrenal (HPA) axis and involves a cascade of stress hormones that produce physiological changes in the body to help us survive.

It works like this: When the body perceives a threat, the brain immediately sets off an alarm system in the body. The sympathetic nervous system kicks into gear, releasing fight, flight, or freeze hormones, including adrenaline. Adrenaline causes the heart rate to increase; air passages to dilate; blood to move to the heart, brain, lungs, and muscles; and mental alertness to increase. All of these physiological changes help us physically react in moments of danger.

Seconds after the sympathetic nervous system is activated, the HPA axis is stimulated. The area of the brain called the hypothalamus sends a signal to the pituitary gland, which releases a hormone to signal the adrenal glands to release the stress hormone cortisol.

Cortisol helps provide an immediate boost of energy by releasing stored glucose into the bloodstream and keeping your blood pressure elevated. It inhibits functions that are considered unimportant during a crisis, including digestion, libido, reproduction, and detoxification. Cortisol enhances and prolongs the fight, flight, or freeze response.

In most cases, when the perceived danger or stressor is gone, this system quiets back down, and the body quickly recovers from the stress. But what happens when stress is ongoing or chronic? Chronic stress can stem from feeling unhappy or overwhelmed with your job, financial worries, the weight of political conflicts, facing discrimination or racism, or—your reason for reading this book—the fear and frustration around trying to get pregnant. Chronic stress leads to chronically elevated stress hormones, particularly cortisol, which can result in anxiety, fatigue, digestive issues, trouble sleeping, weight gain, decreased immune function, and difficulty with memory and focus . . . none of which are good when you are trying to conceive.

The Stress Response and Reproductive Hormones

In Chapter 2, we discussed how the intricate hormonal dance between the brain and ovaries (known as the hypothalamic-pituitary-ovarian, or HPO, axis) is essential for developing healthy eggs, ovulation, and supporting the early stages of pregnancy. If you are an ovulating person, have you ever had a stressful stretch of time (such as a new job, moving, planning your wedding, or the loss of a loved one), and then your period was late the following month? This could be attributed to stress hormones, particularly cortisol, affecting the HPO axis and resulting in a delay in ovulation. When the adrenals release excess cortisol, the hypothalamus may respond by decreasing the amount of hormone it sends to the pituitary. This causes the pituitary to produce lower levels of FSH and LH, which then decreases the production of estrogen, progesterone, and testosterone, resulting in a delay in ovulation.

Increased stress hormones also affect the sperm factor. The same hormonal cascade influencing egg production and ovulation is at play with sperm production. In this case, lower levels of FSH and LH lead to a decrease in testosterone and sperm production in the testes.

Testosterone isn't just for sperm production and muscle growth. It's needed for a healthy libido. Testosterone is the sex hormone with the greatest impact on sex drive for all genders. So when your brain sends stress signals and decreases production of testosterone, it decreases your desire for physical intimacy. Additionally, the release of adrenaline from the sympathetic nervous system causes a decrease of blood flow to the penis, making it difficult for a sperm-producing partner to achieve or maintain an erection.

Herbs to Support a Healthy Stress Response

Fortunately, there are lifestyle modifications and herbal remedies that will help support the body's stress response system so that your hormones return to baseline levels.

Adaptogens

Adaptogens are a group of herbs that help the body adapt to stress, mainly by regulating stress-related hormones and neurotransmitters. Adaptogens are safe and will help boost your body's resistance to stress, have a normalizing effect (meaning they can increase or decrease the body's production of certain hormones depending on what is needed), and work by supporting the HPA axis.

When working with people trying to conceive, the three most common adaptogens I find myself reaching for are eleuthero, reishi, and schisandra. These herbs work best with consistent and regular use over several weeks.

Herbal Nervines

An herbal nervine is an herb that has calming and soothing effects on the nervous system. Herbal nervines ease frayed nerves, lift a gloomy mood, and help us chill out. They are relaxing without making you sleepy. Nervines are wonderful to pair with adaptogens. While adaptogens work on the HPA axis over time, these nervines have a more immediate effect. It's common to notice a shift in mood or anxiety before you finish drinking a cup of nervine tea. Like all herbs, each nervine has its own personality and should be chosen to support your specific needs.

Chamomile

Chamomile (*Matricaria chamomilla*) is often overlooked as a common tea, but don't underestimate the medicinal powers of this familiar herb! It is a powerful nervine and boasts a long list of herbal benefits, such as reducing inflammation, fighting viruses and bacteria, decreasing anxiety, improving digestion, and supporting sleep.

Powerful Support for PMS

Studies have shown that chamomile relieves menstrual cramps just as well as (or better than, in some studies) nonsteroidal, anti-inflammatory drugs (such as ibuprofen) and is effective in reducing the emotional symptoms associated with PMS.[3] Even modest amounts were more effective than a placebo at relieving anxiety and depression in one clinical study.[4] Studies used both capsules and tea, but when using tea the typical dose was 2 cups per day.

I find chamomile helpful for PMS mood disturbances, anxiety, or irritability, particularly in people who have a "nervous stomach." Chamomile helps people switch from the tense, sympathetic nervous system mode, or stress mode, to the more relaxed parasympathetic mode. Many people find chamomile's calming effects are not too sedating to use during the day, but they are strong enough to help with insomnia in the evening.

To fully enjoy a medicinally potent and delicious cup of chamomile tea, skip the powdery tea bags and try a high-quality, organic, loose-leaf chamomile tea. You will notice most of the flowers are still whole, and the aroma is full and complex. Chamomile is also available as a tincture or capsule.

Chamomile is generally safe for most people but can cause allergic reactions in some individuals. People are more likely to react negatively if they're allergic to related plants, such as ragweed, chrysanthemums, marigolds, or daisies.

Typical Dosage Ranges

Tea: 1 tablespoon of dried chamomile per cup of tea, 2–4 cups per day

Tincture: 4–6 mL, two or three times per day

Capsules: 250–500 mg, two or three times per day

Cup of Calm Tea

This soothing blend combines chamomile's anxiety-relieving benefits with the mood-boosting effects of lemon balm, while a pinch of lavender adds a lovely flavor and an extra calming layer.

½ tablespoon dried chamomile flowers

½ tablespoon dried lemon balm

   Pinch of dried lavender flower buds

8 ounces boiling water

Place the herbs in a mesh tea basket in a mug. Cover the herbs with the boiling water and steep for 5-20 minutes. Steeping the tea for 5 minutes will bring out the flavor and medicinal qualities, while steeping longer will bring out more of chamomile's bitter flavors (helpful for digestion) and make a stronger medicinal tea. Remove the tea basket and enjoy.

Combining adaptogens and nervines is a powerful way to support yourself through stressful times, particularly when feeling drained, overwhelmed, scared, anxious, or disappointed . . . feelings often associated with infertility. Fertility journeys can be hard, and herbs help us cope with hard things.

Eleuthero

Eleuthero (*Eleutherococcus senticosus*) is one of the most researched herbs and was the first plant identified as an adaptogen by Soviet scientists in the 1950s. Since then, thousands of studies have shown that eleuthero root can help reduce stress and fatigue, increase mental alertness and performance, improve concentration, increase energy and stamina, improve athletic performance, and enhance immunity.

Lowers Cortisol Levels

So how does it work in relation to fertility? Eleuthero has stress-relieving effects on the HPA axis, reducing levels of the stress hormone the hypothalamus sends to the pituitary gland (called corticotropin-releasing hormone) and dampening the fight, flight, or freeze response in the sympathetic nervous system by lowering noradrenaline.[5] This in turn lowers the stress hormone cascade overall, resulting in lower cortisol levels.

Eleuthero, in combination with lifestyle interventions, is particularly useful for people who are overworked, overextended, and exhausted or who feel "burnt out." A side benefit is that over time, eleuthero reduces the incidence of cold, flu, and other common illnesses.

Eleuthero is a slightly warming, moistening, and semi-stimulating herb. Most people find this herb energizing, not overly stimulating, but if you are sensitive to stimulants you may want to start slow and see how it affects you.

Eleuthero is available in capsule, tincture, powder, or dried herb form. It's also becoming more popular to find eleuthero in coffee and coffee alternative blends, but I recommend a capsule or tincture for my clients to maintain a consistent medicinal dosage.

Typical Dosage Ranges

Tea: 1–2 teaspoons of dried herb in 10–12 ounces of boiling water, 1–3 cups per day

Powder: 2–3 g (1 teaspoon equals about 2.5 g) per day

Tincture: 4–6 mL, two or three times per day

Capsules: 250–500 mg, two to four times per day

Lemon Balm

Lemon balm (*Melissa officinalis*) is revered by herbalists for its mood-elevating effects. Enjoyed as a tea, it can feel like sunshine in a mug! Side benefits of this mint-family plant are that it is high in antioxidants, fights common viruses, is good for digestion, and helps with mental focus.

A recent review of clinical trials confirmed what herbalists have seen first-hand—lemon balm is effective in improving anxiety and depressive symptoms, particularly when taken in the moment.[6] Lemon balm can work quickly, quelling anxiety and lifting mood within an hour of ingesting. Simply smelling the fresh lemon balm plant can brighten your day. I particularly like lemon balm for people who are feeling down, angry, or anxious or who experience premenstrual irritability.

Lemon balm is an aromatic herb that makes a delicious tea alone or combined with other herbs (check out my Cup of Calm Tea recipe on page 113). Tincture or capsules are also available.

Typical Dosage Ranges

Tea: 1 tablespoon of dried lemon balm per cup of tea, 2–4 cups per day
Tincture: 4–6 mL, two or three times per day
Capsules: 250–500 mg, two to four times per day

Simple Lemon Balm Tea

1 tablespoon dried lemon balm
8 ounces boiling water

Place the lemon balm in a mesh tea basket in a mug. Add the boiling water. Cover and steep for 10-15 minutes (or longer!). Remove the tea basket and enjoy. You can add fresh lemon slices after steeping if desired.

Cold Lemon Balm Water

If you have access to fresh lemon balm (an incredibly easy-to-grow plant in most regions), simply cut a large handful of the fresh plant before it flowers and place in a pitcher. Fill with cold water and drink throughout the day (the herbal water will last for 24 hours when refrigerated).

Reishi

Reishi (*Ganoderma lucidum*) mushroom has a long history of use in traditional Chinese medicine (TCM), where it's known as the "mushroom of immortality" for its profound effect on health and longevity. As an adaptogen, reishi helps support the immune system, modulate the stress response, build calm energy, and soothe nerves.

Reishi stands out for its calming effects on the nervous system. In TCM, reishi is often used to help support the shen. Shen can be described as a person's mind or consciousness and emotional balance. Disturbances in shen can show up as anxiety, insomnia, bad dreams, moodiness, confusion, irritability, and poor memory.

Supports Emotional Resilience

When facing a personal challenge or setback, it's normal to get caught up in negative emotions. Reishi supports emotional resilience and your ability to navigate adversity. It's your herbal ally for staying emotionally strong and adaptable, keeping your mental well-being in check.

I find this warming and drying mushroom most helpful for people who tend to feel anxious, nervous, or forgetful or have disturbed sleep. Reishi's calming and relaxing properties make this a wonderful herb during your fertility journey and throughout life.

Reishi mushroom powder can be made as a tea or blended into warm beverages and coffees. Tinctures or capsules are also a convenient way to incorporate into your day.

Typical Dosage Ranges

Powder: 1–4 g (1 teaspoon equals about 3 g) per day
Tincture: 4–6 mL, two or three times per day
Capsules: 250–500 mg, two to four times per day

Schisandra Berry

Schisandra (*Schisandra chinensis*) has a long history of use in TCM to increase vitality, mental clarity, libido, and sexual function. Like other adaptogens, schisandra helps the body adapt to stress. It has a calming effect on the nervous system, improves energy and focus, helps relieve anxiety, and softens anger.

Schisandra shines for its benefits in the liver. One of the liver's main jobs is to metabolize and clear toxins and wastes from the bloodstream. Medications, environmental toxins, and even excess hormones are safely eliminated from the body through the liver. Schisandra increases liver detoxifying enzymes, which helps the liver do its job to support gentle, daily detoxification.

Helps Release Anger

According to TCM, anger is closely related to the liver. The belief is that when the liver is not functioning optimally, emotions can build up and we feel angry, frustrated, or anxious. I find schisandra particularly good at releasing anger and increasing feelings of joy. Who couldn't use more joy in their life, especially when trying to start a family? Schisandra is also helpful when stress is affecting the ability to concentrate, focus, or just get work done. Schisandra can help lower cortisol levels so we feel less stressed out and improve focus and cognition, helping us get back to the task at hand.

The Chinese word for schisandra means "five flavors" in English, so named because it is the only berry that tastes simultaneously salty, sour, bitter, pungent, and sweet. The flavor is quite unique! The dried berry can be enjoyed as a tea (often blended with other herbs or honey to soften the sourness), tincture, or capsule or even eaten straight (get ready for the flavor burst!).

Caution: Because schisandra increases liver detoxifying enzymes, it may interact with some medications. Check with a professional before trying. Do not take it once you are pregnant, as it may stimulate uterine contractions.

Typical Dosage Ranges

Tea: 1 teaspoon of dried schisandra berry per cup of tea, 2–3 cups per day
Powder: 1–3 g per day
Tincture: 4–6 mL, two or three times per day
Capsules: 250–500 mg, two or three times per day
Dried berries: about 10 berries per day

Schisandra Berry Hibiscus Tea

1 teaspoon dried schisandra berries
2 teaspoons dried hibiscus flowers
8 ounces boiling water
Honey

Combine the schisandra and hibiscus in a mesh tea basket in a mug. Add the boiling water. Cover and steep for 10-15 minutes. Remove the tea basket, add honey to taste, and enjoy. The tea can also be served cold, over ice with a splash of seltzer.

Getting Better Sleep

While getting a good night's rest is an important part of managing stress, lack of sleep does more than just make us tired and cranky. It can increase oxidative stress, which, as we know, is the enemy of both healthy sperm and healthy eggs. Healthy sleep helps regulate the hormones important to reproduction, and disruptions in our slumber negatively affect fertility.

Essential for Producing Fertility Hormones

Sleep affects the production of the key fertility hormones estrogen, progesterone, LH, and FSH. Proper sleep is critical to keep these hormones in balance. Long-term insomnia may directly affect the release of the hormone that triggers ovulation (LH), resulting in irregular cycles.

LH and FSH are also crucial for the production of testosterone and sperm in the testes. Testosterone plays an important role in libido, erectile function, and sperm health. Getting only 5 hours of sleep can decrease testosterone production by about 15 percent, which is equivalent to the decline a person would experience aging naturally over 15 years. Compounding matters, low testosterone may get in the way of a good night's sleep, making it harder to fall asleep and stay asleep. It becomes a vicious cycle—the less you sleep the lower your testosterone production falls, and the lower testosterone levels make it harder for you to sleep.

Another important fertility hormone is leptin, which regulates the menstrual cycle and affects ovulation. Research shows that getting less than 7–8 hours of sleep has been associated with reduced leptin levels the following day,[7] and disturbances in this hormone have been linked to irregular menstrual cycles and poor egg quality.[8]

LEPTIN AND SATIETY

Leptin controls your feeling of fullness after eating. Also referred to as the satiety hormone, leptin sends signals to your brain that you have enough food, specifically fat, helping you feel satiated. You may have noticed that after a poor night of sleep, you make less-healthy food choices or tend to overindulge the next day. That's your brain responding to lower leptin levels, directing you to eat more and signaling your cells to hold on to fat.

Tips for Getting Better Sleep

Studies suggest we need at least 7 hours of sleep per night, but many of us need more. Here are some simple tips to help you get the sleep you need.

Get into a routine. Go to bed and wake up at the same time. Keep this schedule 7 days a week—yes, even on weekends!

Get outside in the morning. Ten minutes of natural sunlight in the morning will boost melatonin (a hormone that helps us sleep) that evening.

Stop eating at night. Avoid large meals and snacks before bedtime. Eating before bed and eating late at night may help you fall asleep initially, but when blood sugar crashes in the middle of the night, cortisol levels rise and melatonin production diminishes.

No coffee or tea, please. Avoid caffeine after noon, or entirely if you are sensitive to caffeine.

Limit alcohol. Stick to one serving in the evening, or eliminate altogether; consider swapping out your evening glass of wine with a cup of chamomile or lemon balm tea.

Unplug yourself. Turn off all electronic devices (blue light affects melatonin) at least 1 hour before bedtime, including smartphones, tablets, and the television.

Chill out. Dim the lights and find some relaxing activities like meditation or reading.

Exercise earlier in the day. While exercise is good for healthy sleep–wake cycles, try to avoid late-night exercise, which can be overly stimulating.

Cool it down. Keep the bedroom temperature between 60 and 65°F (16 and 18°C).

Keep it dark. Use blackout shades, curtains, or an eye mask to keep all light out of the bedroom. Even relatively dim light—about the equivalent of a hallway light—can have a profound effect on sleep.

Herbs to Support Healthy Sleep

Coupling herbs with healthy sleep habits is a powerful way to break the sleep–stress cycle and get back on track for a consistent and restorative night's rest. Making a cup of herbal tea after dinner is a great way to wind down from your day and tell your body it's time to relax. Tinctures are also a convenient way to take herbs. Lemon balm and chamomile, the nervine herbs we discussed previously in this chapter, are very good for helping you get a better night's rest. Below are a few more herbs specifically for sleep.

Ashwagandha

A discussion about sleep wouldn't be complete without ashwagandha (*Withania somnifera*). The second part of its Latin name, *somnifera*, means "sleep-inducing." But it isn't a sedating herb, so it won't make you sleepy. On the contrary, ashwagandha works to build energy and vitality when taken regularly. Its impact on sleep happens slowly, over time, by improving the stress response, lowering cortisol levels in the evening, and raising cortisol in the morning. This supports your natural circadian rhythm so you can fall asleep easier, stay asleep throughout the night, and wake feeling rested. Ashwagandha also increases GABA levels in the brain. GABA is a neurotransmitter that calms your nervous system down, so you don't become overly anxious or afraid, and helps you fall asleep and stay asleep. Ashwagandha is ideal for people who feel anxious or tired and struggle to get a good night's sleep.

Warning: Ashwagandha is part of the nightshade family, so if you react negatively to nightshade plants, you may want to avoid it or start with very small doses to see how you feel. In my experience, most people with nightshade sensitivities can tolerate ashwagandha without issue.

Typical Dosage Ranges

Powder: 2–6 g (1 teaspoon equals about 4 g) per day

Tincture: 4–6 mL, two or three times per day

Capsules: 250–500 mg, two to four times per day

Recipes: Maca Nut Butter Balls (see page 99), Golden Milk (see page 94; but made with ½ teaspoon ashwagandha), Chocolate Banana Almond Smoothie (see page 96)

Passionflower

Passionflower (*Passiflora incarnata*) is a sedating nervine that helps you fall asleep, eases anxiety, and decreases agitation. It is for those times when you put your head on the pillow and suddenly the mental chatter starts . . . and won't turn off. If you tend to overthink or worry and it's getting in the way of sleep, passionflower is a wonderful herb to try. It blends well in teas, but many people find keeping a tincture bottle on their nightstand an easy way to reach for this herb on a restless night.

Typical Dosage Ranges

Tea: 1 tablespoon of dried passionflower per cup of tea, 2–4 cups per day
Tincture: 1–8 mL, two or three times per day
Capsules: 250–500 mg, one or two times per day

Skullcap

Skullcap (*Scutellaria lateriflora*) is a calming, sedating herb that helps you unwind and relax, especially when you're feeling tense, agitated, anxious, nervous, and overstimulated. It helps release physical tension and quiet ruminating thoughts. When taken over time, it can help restore the nervous system so you feel less reactive. The freshly dried herb loses its potency fairly quickly, but the tincture can last for a few years.

Typical Dosage Ranges

Tea: 1 tablespoon of dried skullcap per cup of tea, 2–4 cups per day
Tincture: 1–8 mL, two or three times per day
Capsules: 250–500 mg, one or two times per day

Sleep Tincture

Lemon balm tincture
Passionflower tincture
Skullcap tincture

Combine equal parts of the three herbal tinctures in a clean glass bottle with a dropper top. Shake it up. Take 1-2 mL a few hours before bedtime, then take another 1-2 mL right before bed.

Enhance Fertility with Movement

Movement and exercise are important parts of a healthy lifestyle and can help manage stress and depression. They are also an important part of a holistic fertility plan.

A sedentary lifestyle isn't good for your health, and it isn't good for your fertility. Some experts even say that sitting is the new smoking. Did you know that after just 30 minutes of sitting, your metabolism and lymphatic detox system start to slow down? And after 4 hours of sitting, your blood sugar levels increase to a level that the body perceives as stress.

Regular movement helps counter the effects of the sedentary modern world—from sitting at a desk for hours at a time to driving in a car to lounging on the couch. It can help improve blood flow to the pelvic region, ensuring that reproductive organs receive an adequate supply of oxygen and nutrients. Regular exercise can help alleviate stress and depression. Studies have shown that exercise alone works as well as antidepressants.[9]

How Much Exercise Is Safe?

But how much exercise is considered safe when trying to conceive? The general consensus is that 30–60 minutes of exercise daily is fine, but more than 60 minutes per day has an increased risk of ovulation disruption.[10] Excessive exercise can send a signal to the brain that it isn't safe to reproduce and affects ovulation in some people.

With this in mind, the goal is to find the balance that's right for you. What is considered "moderate" exercise for one person may be "strenuous" for another. Do the "talk test" (talk while you are exercising and find the level where you do not feel exhausted or depleted) to find your ideal level.

If you are new to exercise or just getting back into it, try some more gentle forms of movement, such as yoga, Pilates, walking, tai chi, strength training, swimming, or dancing. These activities can be a great way to safely ease into a routine that can help support overall health and wellness. Even something as simple as taking stretch breaks throughout your day can be helpful for getting the blood flowing.

If you sit for work, try the Pomodoro Technique for focused work time and built-in movement breaks. It works like this: Using a timer, set a 25-minute block of time for focused work, immediately followed by a 5-minute break to move around—stretch, chair exercises, or a short walk. Repeat this cycle throughout the day, with longer breaks as needed. Many people find this helps with focus, creativity, and meeting their daily movement goals.

Mindfulness and Meditation

Over the past 15 years, research has confirmed that mindfulness-based practices like meditation are the best medicine for modern living. Meditation doesn't just help us relax—it actually changes our brains. It builds brain volume in the parts associated with working memory, decision-making, self-relevance, learning, emotional regulation, empathy, and compassion. Even more amazing, meditation shrinks the amygdala, the brain's center for anxiety, fear, and stress. These changes have been confirmed on brain scans after 8 weeks of a regular meditation practice of just 20 minutes per day.

Flip the Stress Switch

When used during times of stress, meditation is a way to quickly flip the switch, moving our bodies from stress (sympathetic response) into relaxation (parasympathetic response) and all the chemical, physical, hormonal, and metabolic changes that go along with these responses. Meditation, quite literally, hacks your brain and nervous system so you can weather life's ups and downs feeling less reactive, stressed, angry, sad, and agitated. The best part is that everyone has access to it—from anywhere—for free!

What's good for the egg is often good for the sperm, and meditation is no exception. One study found that just 21 days of a yoga-based meditation practice resulted in a significant improvement in sperm count and motility and a decline in oxidative DNA damage.[11] Mindfulness-based techniques have also been shown to effectively treat low libido.[12]

If you think you can't meditate because your mind never settles down, think again. The goal of meditation isn't to "quiet" your mind; it is about deciding *not* to engage with it. It is to notice when thoughts come up (and they will), choose to release them, and come back to your breath. Every time you do this—the act of noticing a thought, letting it go, and coming back—you are flexing your meditation muscle, much like you flex your biceps when you do a curl. That is the purpose of meditation: to keep flexing your "muscle" in order to build a stronger brain over time.

Meditation is about deciding
not to engage with your mind.

Choosing a Style of Meditation

Meditation may be the most important habit you can form . . . next to a daily cup of tea (or three!). Do a quick search on the internet and you'll find several apps and tutorials.

So what type of meditation is the best? The research shows it doesn't really matter. The important thing is to spend time in a state where you are not engaged in your thoughts. Have fun trying different forms of meditation and mindfulness-based practices. Here are a few examples.

Guided meditations. A facilitator leads you through a series of visualizations to promote relaxation, gratitude, or calm.

Mindfulness meditations. Practiced alone or through a facilitator, mindfulness meditations focus on awareness of the present moment, observing thoughts and sensations without judgment.

Mantra-based meditations. This type of meditation involves repeating a specific word, phrase, or sound to focus the mind.

Breathing exercises. One example is four-by-four breathing: Inhale four counts, hold four counts, exhale four counts, hold four counts. Repeat three or four times.

Mindful walking. Walk in silence, paying attention to all five senses.

Coloring books. Pick up a set of colored pencils, markers, or crayons and lose yourself.

JACK AND EMILY'S STORIES
Managing Stress

While focusing on getting pregnant, it's easy to overlook the importance of managing stress, yet supporting the body and supporting the mind are equally important on this journey.

JACK

As we mentioned in Chapter 8, Jack was already taking ashwagandha to help with sperm motility and morphology, anxiety, and sleep. We also decreased his caffeine intake by swapping his afternoon coffees for green tea. Here are the lifestyle changes we added to Jack's protocol.

Jack committed to putting his phone on the charger 1 hour before going to bed. The charger was relocated outside the bedroom so he wasn't tempted to scroll before going to sleep.

He and his partner agreed on an ideal sleep schedule. They held each other accountable when one wanted to "watch one more episode" or "finish up a quick thing for work" and stuck to their bedtime schedule. On weekends, they resisted the temptation to sleep in and instead woke up together, enjoying a leisurely start to their day.

Jack agreed to try four-by-four breathing every morning, once after lunch, and just before bed. After a few weeks, he noticed he was looking forward to what he called his "nervous system reset."

EMILY

Emily's main goals were to support egg quality and decrease period pain. Using an overnight infusion, ginger tea, or capsules, and setting a timer to keep her moving through her workday, we had made progress, but the stress of life and trying to conceive was starting to take a toll. It was time to add some adaptogen support, increase movement, and introduce some mindfulness.

We supported Emily's nervous system with an herbal tincture blend that included eleuthero, schisandra berry, and lemon balm. She took 3 mL in a small amount of water, two times per day.

Emily began a meditation practice using an app on her phone for 10 minutes every morning before leaving for work. The key was to not overthink which app or which meditation, just to pick the one that met her time requirements.

In addition to the short movement breaks throughout her day, we added a 30-minute exercise block to her daily calendar. She could choose to walk, stretch, or do a beginner weight workout.

CHAPTER 10

ENVIRONMENTAL EXPOSURES CAN
SABOTAGE FERTILITY

···

From Pesticides to Plastics

In our modern era, we're surrounded by a staggering number of chemicals and compounds, many of which are lurking under the kitchen sink, on the dinner table, and in your toiletry bag. Despite our bodies' natural detoxification abilities, we haven't adapted to the flood of environmental exposures to combinations of chemicals over time. This has led to a surge in chronic illnesses and an alarming decline in fertility rates.

What Can You Do?

When it comes to learning about environmental exposures, especially those happening within our homes, food, and water, it's normal to feel overwhelmed. Some people feel compelled to eliminate every possible toxin, while others may shrug it off with indifference. However, the key lies in finding balance. We can't do it all, but we also can't do nothing; instead, our focus should be on taking manageable steps in the right direction.

Take control of what you can, while allowing yourself to release the burden of what you can't. It's not about achieving perfection; it's about making meaningful progress. Resist the urge to rush into drastic changes, instead focusing on gradual, sustainable swaps. With time, you'll discover a balanced approach that comes from a place of knowledge and empowerment, not fear.

Reduce Exposure to Pesticides

Eating fruits and vegetables that have high amounts of pesticide residues—such as strawberries, spinach, kale, or grapes—decreases a person's chances of conceiving. Studies show that pesticides can impact egg and sperm quality as well as overall fertility. In one study, eating fruits and vegetables with high levels of pesticide residues was associated with 49 percent lower total sperm count and 32 percent lower sperm morphology than found in people with the lowest intake of pesticides.[1]

In another study, people undergoing fertility treatment were separated into two groups: One ate high amounts of organic fruits and veggies and the other ate conventional (nonorganic) fruits and veggies. The nonorganic group had 18 percent fewer pregnancies.[2]

Eat Organic Foods Whenever Possible

The term *organic* refers to the way agricultural products are grown and processed. While the regulations vary from country to country, in the United States, organic crops must be grown without the use of synthetic pesticides, bioengineered genes (GMOs), petroleum-based fertilizers, and sewage sludge–based fertilizers (Code of Federal Regulations, 2021).

Eating organic foods makes a difference. In just 1 week of eating mostly organic foods, the level of pesticides detected in a person's urine is reduced by nearly 90 percent.[3]

AVOID THE DIRTY DOZEN

Need help choosing which produce should be organic and which is okay to eat conventionally grown? Check out the Environmental Working Group's Dirty Dozen and Clean 15 annual report.

The EWG's 2024 Dirty Dozen
These have the most pesticide residue, so choose organic.

- Strawberries
- Spinach
- Kale, collard, and mustard greens
- Grapes
- Peaches
- Pears
- Nectarines
- Apples
- Bell and hot peppers
- Cherries
- Blueberries
- Green beans

The EWG's 2024 Clean 15
Conventionally grown produce on this list has the lowest level of pesticides.

- Avocados
- Sweet corn
- Pineapples
- Onions
- Papayas
- Sweet peas (frozen)
- Asparagus
- Honeydew melons
- Kiwifruit
- Cabbage
- Watermelons
- Mushrooms
- Mangos
- Sweet potatoes
- Carrots

Prioritize produce. If cost or access is an issue, prioritize organic produce, as fruits and vegetables are often heavily sprayed with pesticides. Check out the Environmental Working Group's (EWG) Dirty Dozen and Clean 15 lists (see facing page) to help you decide which conventionally grown produce has the highest levels of pesticides and should be avoided unless organic and which has lower pesticide levels.

Unwashed produce can have even more residues, so it's a good idea to wash everything before you eat it. Just remember that washing or peeling your produce isn't enough to remove all pesticides.

Then focus on animal products and packaged foods. Organic dairy products are next, followed by organic, grass-fed, pasture-raised sourced animal products such as eggs, beef, chicken, and pork. While organic grains and packaged foods are beneficial, they can be less of a priority if the budget is tight. When it comes to fish, opt for wild-caught varieties over farm-raised. Wild-caught fish generally have lower levels of contaminants and higher nutritional value. Beware of marketing claims: There's no such thing as wild-caught, organic fish. Only farmed fish can be organic, and wild-caught is still preferable. By strategically allocating your resources, you can prioritize organic foods for optimal health and still stay within your budget constraints.

Reduce Exposure to Bisphenols

Bisphenol chemicals are everywhere—they're some of the most commonly produced chemicals globally and are found in countless products. Bisphenol A (BPA), the most researched of the bisphenols, is used in items from plastic water bottles and food containers to cash register receipts and linings inside canned foods and drinks. Over the past 20 years, scientific knowledge of the effects of BPA has grown exponentially and the conclusion is clear: Even small amounts of BPA can mess with your hormone-sensitive organs and are related to a wide range of health issues.

Endocrine-Disrupting BPA

BPA is an endocrine disruptor, meaning it binds to hormone receptors and disrupts the way reproductive hormones like estrogen and testosterone work. BPA has been linked to cancer, heart disease, and fertility issues.

Research shows that BPA negatively impacts sperm health. One study revealed that individuals exposed to high levels of BPA at work had lower sperm count and motility.[4] Another study found that people going through IVF who had higher levels of BPA also had lower sperm count, sperm concentration, and sperm vitality.[5]

BPA doesn't just affect sperm—it also affects egg quality and the success of fertility treatments like IVF. Research on IVF cycles has found that exposure to BPA is linked to lower estrogen levels, which can mean fewer eggs are available for retrieval. Additionally, it's been associated with a higher chance of implantation failure, reducing the probability of pregnancy and increasing the risk of miscarriage.

So how do we end up with BPA in our system? Remember the old adage "You are what you eat"? Well, the same goes for BPA exposure. BPA seeps into food, especially when it's hot or when the food is acidic.

ARE "BPA-FREE" PRODUCTS BETTER?

As consumer concerns over BPA increased, the US FDA began to get on board by doing things like banning the sale of baby bottles containing BPA in 2012. Companies started switching to similar chemicals like bisphenol S (BPS) and bisphenol F (BPF), and proudly advertising their new "BPA-Free" products. But here's the catch: These substitutes are just as hormone-disrupting as BPA. In fact, some research suggests that BPS, a common replacement for BPA, might be even worse for our reproductive systems.[6] So just because something says "BPA-Free" doesn't mean it's all good.

Strategies to Reduce Exposure to Bisphenols

- Swap out plastic containers in favor of glass or stainless steel.

- Never reheat food in a plastic container.

- Reduce the use of canned foods.

- Swap coffee pod systems (most plastic coffee pods contain BPA) or choose nonplastic pods.

- Limit packaged foods in the diet.

- Skip plastic water bottles and large water jug dispensers.

- Reduce exposure to aluminum beverage cans, including seltzer, soda, and beer.

- Avoid handling paper receipts and other thermal paper, as BPA can be absorbed through the skin.

Reduce Exposure to Phthalates

One thing that cologne, body wash, air fresheners, scented deodorants, and takeout food containers all have in common is a group of chemicals called phthalates. They are used in plastics to make them soft and flexible and in artificial fragrances to make the scent last longer. Phthalates, like bisphenols, are known hormone disruptors. Exposure to phthalates has been linked to early puberty, breast and skin cancers, allergies, asthma, obesity, insulin resistance, diabetes, endometriosis, and fertility issues.

Lower Sperm Count and Compromised Ovarian Function

Several studies have found that phthalates have negative effects on sperm. They've been linked to lower sperm count and motility, lower testosterone levels,[7] an increased time to pregnancy, and increased risk of miscarriage.[8]

Other studies have suggested that phthalates can affect ovarian function. Patients going through IVF with higher levels of phthalates had fewer eggs at retrieval, lower fertilization rates, and lower implantation rates, leading to a decrease in the chances of getting pregnant through IVF treatments. Phthalates may also play a role in developing premature ovarian insufficiency and endometriosis.[9]

Strategies to Reduce Exposure to Phthalates

Avoid artificial fragrances in personal products. This is one of the most effective ways to decrease phthalate exposure. One study tested the urine of pregnant people and found those who used perfume had phthalate concentrations 167 percent higher than nonusers.[10]

Look for and avoid the ingredient "fragrance" in personal care products. This is a big task, but well worth the time and money. Start by auditing the products you use every day—shampoo, conditioner, body wash, soap, perfume, cologne, deodorant, aftershave, moisturizer, makeup, and nail polish, to name a few. If "fragrance" is listed as an ingredient, it likely contains phthalates. Begin replacing your products with ones that don't list "fragrance" (or "parfum"/"perfume") as an ingredient—choose instead ones that use essential oils. The EWG's Skin Deep Cosmetics Database is a great place to start researching cleaner personal care products.

HOW TO SPOT PHTHALATES: DECODING LABELS

Phthalates are not easy to spot because they are rarely listed as an ingredient on labels. Why? Because the FDA does not require the listing of the individual components that make up fragrances. Any time you see the ingredient "fragrance" listed on a label, assume phthalates are present. Unscented products are not necessarily phthalate-free because they often contain masking fragrances. Unfortunately, the term *natural fragrances* isn't regulated, so anything that lists this could also include phthalates. The only way to know for sure is if the company lists the specific fragrance ingredients.

Here are some terms to look for on labels:

- Fragrance
- Parfum or perfume
- Phthalate

- Diethyl phthalate (DEP)
- Dimethyl phthalate (DMP)
- Dibutyl phthalate (DBP)

Choose organic, fragrance-free tampons and pads. Researchers have found endocrine-disrupting chemicals in menstrual products, which are absorbed through the highly permeable vaginal and vulvar tissue. The specific chemicals found include phthalates, volatile organic compounds, parabens, environmental phenols, fragrance chemicals, dioxins, and dioxin-like compounds. Choosing organic, fragrance-free products can lead you to safer alternatives, as well as searching on the EWG's Skin Deep Cosmetics Database.

Ditch your home air fresheners, scented candles, and scented trash bags. Again, scan the ingredient list for "fragrance." You can find safer alternatives that use essential oils, which are phthalate-free.

Clean up your cleaning products. For cleaning products, it can be harder to find ingredient lists, but the EWG's Guide to Healthy Cleaning is a helpful resource.

Limit exposure to soft plastics. Common products include shower curtains, inflatable pool floats, plastic toys, disposable food storage containers, and raincoats. Choose more natural materials when possible.

HOW TO AVOID MICROPLASTICS IN TEA BAGS

The bad news is that some tea bags contain tiny plastic particles that can seep into your tea. But here's the good news: There are plenty of options available for a safer brew.

Certain types of tea bags release millions of plastic bits into your drink. When hot water meets plastic in tea bags, it can lead to the release of microplastics and nanoplastics into your tea. In fact, a single cup can contain billions of these tiny particles, way more than what you'd find in other foods and drinks. The highest levels of microplastics were found in the tea bags that resemble silky pyramids, but some paper tea bags use plastic sealants and coatings as well.

Here's how to brew a safer cup of tea.

Pick the right bag. Look for tea brands that guarantee their tea bags are free from harmful chemicals like BPA, phthalates, polypropylene, polyethylene terephthalate (PET), plant-based polylactic acid (PLA), and epichlorohydrin. Opt for tea bags made from organic hemp, unbleached cotton, or plant fibers for a safer alternative.

Go loose. Consider using loose-leaf teas and steep them using a stainless steel mesh strainer or a French press.

Choose organic. This will minimize pesticide exposure, but remember that being organic doesn't always mean the tea bag is plastic-free. Plastic is a separate issue that organic certifications don't address.

Filter Your Water

Most of us don't think about the water we drink. We know water is essential for good health and we try to drink at least eight glasses every day. But what if our water isn't as pure as we think? If you are drinking water straight out of the tap, it may contain more contaminants than you realize. Contaminants from industrial dumping (legal or illegal), lead, "forever chemicals" known as PFAS, agricultural pesticides, disinfection chemicals, and pharmaceuticals top the list of toxins showing up in the water.

Consider the following:

- 77 million Americans—that's nearly 1 in 4 people—drink tap water that is in violation of the Safe Drinking Water Act because of excess contamination.

- 5,300 US water systems are in violation of lead rules, including failure to properly test water for lead, failure to report contamination to residents, and failure to treat water properly to avoid lead contamination.

- A National Public Radio investigation reported more than 3,000 cases around the United States where lead levels were double that of Flint, Michigan. There is a strong scientific consensus that any amount of lead exposure during childhood is harmful.

- Research from the EWG shows that the majority of Americans are exposed to PFAS in their drinking water, frequently exceeding the recommended safe limits. The persistent "forever chemicals" are linked to hormone disruption, diminished sperm health, prolonged time to conception, some cancers, and various other health issues.

- Almost 90 percent of tap water sampled by the US Department of Agriculture (USDA) had traces of the herbicide atrazine, often at concentrations higher than what the federal law allows. It is also found in well water, as atrazine leaches into groundwater and then into the well. Atrazine is a hormone-disrupting chemical linked to an increased risk of miscarriage, birth defects, poor sperm quality, menstrual problems, and an elevated risk of breast and prostate cancers.

- The Centers for Disease Control and Prevention is calling contaminated drinking water "one of the most seminal public health challenges of the coming decades."

Is Bottled Water Better?

Considering these alarming facts, let's discuss bottled water. While many view it as a safer alternative, the truth is less reassuring. Surprisingly, a study in 2009 found that half of all bottled water is simply tap water sourced directly from local municipalities!

Another significant concern regarding bottled water is the plastic packaging itself, whether it's the small, single-use bottles or the large jugs commonly delivered to homes or workplaces. Most single-use water bottles are made of a type of plastic called polyethylene terephthalate (PET). Several studies have found that PET plastic bottles can release hormone-disrupting chemicals into the water. Plus, a study in 2024 found that bottled water contains not just PET but also six other types of plastic bits, called nanoplastics, in much higher amounts than previously thought.[11] And let's not forget about the environmental impact all these plastic bottles have, creating tons of waste that's harmful to our planet.

CHRIS'S STORY
Daily Choices to Boost Sperm Count

Chris and his partner met with me after learning that Chris had received discouraging news about his low sperm count, morphology, and mobility. Their fertility clinic said their only option was to use IVF—in other words, natural or IUI procedures wouldn't get them pregnant. On top of that, Chris likely wouldn't have enough healthy swimmers from only one sample to use at egg retrieval. The plan was to bank and freeze several samples leading up to the procedure and combine them for the best chance of fertilization.

During our initial meeting, I learned two critical pieces of information: (1) Chris commuted 1 hour each way, every day, to his job. It was the middle of winter, and he always turned on the heated seat in his car. (2) He loved his cologne and never skipped a day without a spritz.

Here's how we supported Chris and his sperm.

Herbs. Ashwagandha, green tea, and turmeric
Supplements. Multivitamin, CoQ10, and omega-3s
Reduced exposures. We swapped cologne for a natural brand free of synthetic fragrances. Chris stopped using heated car seats.

Three months later, Chris underwent a follow-up semen analysis, and to everyone's surprise (except mine), his results showed such significant improvement that the couple received the green light to move forward with the standard IVF process (i.e., no longer needing to take a multitude of semen samples), using a fresh sample at the time of egg retrieval.

While every element of the sperm support protocol likely contributed to this incredible outcome, the impact of heated seats was particularly noteworthy—an aspect often overlooked as a potential sperm saboteur—and a daily dose of phthalates from cologne should not be underestimated. Their first IVF cycle resulted in a successful pregnancy, and Chris and his partner now have a healthy baby.

Test Your Water, Then Filter It

Filtering your tap water offers a safe and reliable solution—but how do you choose the right filter? The official answer is "it depends." It depends on the water quality in your town, if you own or rent your home, and how much money you want to spend. Again, the EWG's Tap Water Database is a great go-to. Searchable by zip code, you can access the water reports for your town so you know what contaminants are typically found in your municipal water. You can also test your own water with companies that offer home test kits.

Countertop filters. Once you know what's in your water, you are ready to select a filter.

A countertop, carbon filter pitcher is the easiest way to filter. Countertop pitchers can filter out most contaminants and come in BPA- and BPS-free containers. Pay attention to the list of contaminants that the pitcher is verified to remove, not just the marketing claims. Some of the most popular countertop pitchers filter very few contaminants. The EWG has a Water Filter Guide that can help you find the right filter for your water and budget.

Under-the-sink filtration systems. Another option is an under-the-sink filtration system. These cost more but are more convenient (no need to refill a pitcher) and provide access to filtered water by just turning on the tap.

Whole-house filters. Another choice is a whole-house filter, but they cost thousands of dollars and may not be necessary for your situation, particularly if you plan to move anytime soon.

It's not just the water you drink. Filtering your shower water is important, too. Chlorine is present in all tap water to disinfect and keep the water free of pathogenic bacteria. Chlorine is a volatile chemical, so it quickly and easily vaporizes. In a hot shower situation, we end up inhaling and absorbing chlorine through our skin in amounts that can exceed what we get from drinking chlorinated water.

Because our skin has its own delicate microbiome, showering or bathing in chlorinated water can exacerbate skin issues like eczema. Chlorine is also a respiratory irritant that can cause or worsen asthma and cause eye and throat irritation. This is even more important when you are pregnant and after the baby is born, when baths are part of the daily routine.

You can filter your shower water using either a showerhead filter or a whole-house system. While whole-house filters can be costly, basic whole-house carbon filters, which you can install yourself, are much cheaper (typically under $100) and are effective for removing chlorine from shower and bath water. However, it's best not to rely on these basic carbon filters for drinking water.

For those with well water, a similar strategy applies. Contaminants such as bacteria, arsenic, and agricultural runoff can seep into well water. Although wells have built-in filtration systems, they may not remove all contaminants. It's a good idea to test your water yearly and consider additional filters if necessary.

Water filtration is a simple way to reduce exposure to potentially harmful contaminants and support your overall health. Resist feeling overwhelmed and choose what feels best for you at this point in your life. You can always make changes down the road.

This one step will have a huge ripple effect for your health and the health of everyone in your home. Think of how often you drink water, tea, or coffee and how many times you shower or bathe. When you have little ones in your home, you may need water for formula, drinking water, and so many baths. This one investment in health will continue to pay off for years to come.

EVERY POSITIVE CHANGE MAKES A DIFFERENCE

When addressing environmental toxins, it's important to remember that progress, not perfection, is the goal. You will never eliminate all toxic exposures from your life, and that's okay. Every step taken to minimize these exposures makes a difference. Your body is remarkably resilient and can handle occasional small exposures; it's the cumulative effect of repeated exposures over time that poses the greatest risk. Celebrate the positive changes you are making to create a healthier body and home for you and your growing family.

Limit Close Contact with Cell Phones and Wireless Laptops

Though this is often dismissed as a myth, studies suggest that keeping a cell phone or laptop close to the groin area negatively affects sperm health. Both devices emit radio frequency electromagnetic radiation (RF-EMR), which has been shown to damage sperm even with "typical" use.

Sperm exposed to RF-EMR levels similar to those from carrying a cell phone in your front pocket or using a laptop on your lap experienced lower motility and viability, along with increased oxidative damage.[12] Moving the phone just 20 inches away from the groin area reduced the amount of sperm damage.[13] So put your phone in your back pocket.

The time spent using your phone also matters. One hour of cell phone radiation had a significant negative impact on sperm motility, DNA fragmentation, and the ability of the sperm to attach and fertilize the egg,[14] while talking less than 1 hour had less damage.[15] The use of a cell phone while charging was associated with a higher percentage of abnormal sperm concentration compared to use of one when it was not charging.[16]

Similar results were seen with WiFi-enabled laptops. Sperm samples exposed to a wireless internet-connected laptop for 4 hours showed a significant decrease in progressive sperm motility and an increase in sperm DNA fragmentation.[17]

The bottom line: There is enough data to suggest taking a precautionary approach to cell phone and laptop use. A simple strategy to minimize the negative effects is to remember that distance and time matters. Whether it's coming from a WiFi laptop or a cell phone, RF-EMR drops off the farther you get from the source, so keep your phone out of your pockets and your laptop off your lap whenever possible.

Avoid Smoking, Vaping, and Cannabis

By now, we all know that smoking is bad for us. Specific to fertility, smoking can prolong the time it takes to conceive; impair the ovaries' ability to produce healthy eggs; reduce sperm count, motility, and morphology; and increase the risk of miscarriage.

Vaping (e-cigarettes), once considered a safer option, is now linked to health risks that are similar to those of cigarettes. A 2023 study found that both vapers and smokers showed high levels of DNA damage, more than double that of non-users,[18] which can negatively affect egg and sperm quality.

Research on cannabis and its effects on fertility is still ongoing, and the findings vary. Some studies indicate a higher likelihood of infertility among ovulating cannabis users, as well as lower sperm quality for sperm-producing users. Cannabis can also interfere with the sperm's ability to bind to the egg, potentially reducing fertilization rates. Until more research is conducted, it's wise to follow the recommendations from the American College of Obstetrics and Gynecologists and the American College of Pediatricians, which advise reducing or abstaining from cannabis use during preconception and pregnancy.

CHAPTER 11

CONDITIONS
THAT AFFECT
FERTILITY

....

How to Support Your Fertility and
When to Seek Medical Advice

If you've gone through this book, made changes to support
your health and fertility, but still feel something's off, this
section is for you. The goal of this chapter is to help you
identify possible issues so you can work with your doctor
for an accurate diagnosis, while also giving you a starting
point to support your health and fertility with natural
strategies. While some issues can improve with nutrition,
herbs, supplements, and lifestyle changes, others will
require medical interventions, medications, and/or fertility
treatments. Regardless of where you land, these strategies
form a solid foundation for achieving the best outcomes,
even alongside medical interventions.

An Overview of Ovulation and Menstruation

Knowing if your periods are irregular will help you better understand your body and your fertility. Often the term *irregular* may refer to a change in what's normal for you. But what does it truly mean to have irregular cycles? Let's explore the characteristics that define irregularity and how they affect your fertility.

In the first half of the menstrual cycle, called the follicular phase, you have your period, and an egg inside a follicle is maturing and getting ready to be released. Ovulation happens when estrogen levels go up, causing an LH surge and the egg to be released. The second half of the menstrual cycle, called the luteal phase, comes after ovulation and is when the uterus is preparing for possible implantation.

So what does a normal menstrual cycle look like?

- Frequency: 24–38 days from the start of one menstrual cycle to the next

- Duration of flow: 4–8 days of bleeding (4–5 days on average), with heaviest bleeding occurring during the first 2–3 days

- The second half: a luteal phase of at least 11 days (12–14 days on average)

- Variability: cycle length varies less than 8 days from one cycle to the next

Irregular cycles describe anything that's not a normal menstrual period. For example:

- Short cycles: less than 24 days from start of one menstrual cycle to the next

- Long cycles: more than 38 days from start of one menstrual cycle to the next

- Short luteal phase: 10 days or less from ovulation to start of period

- Variable cycles: cycle length that varies more than 8 days from one cycle to another

- Missing cycles: not having a period for 3 months

- Heavy flow: needing to change your tampon or pad after less than 2 hours or in the middle of the night, or you see clots the size of a quarter or larger

- Increased duration in flow: bleeding longer than 7 days

- Pain: periods that are accompanied by severe pain, cramping, nausea, or vomiting

- Mid-cycle spotting: bleeding or spotting that happens between periods

Understanding the ins and outs and timing of a person's menstrual cycle offers valuable insights on their road to fertility. When a period is late, irregular, early, completely missing, or very heavy, it's almost always due to changes in ovulation timing. Ovulation, the main event in a menstrual cycle, determines whether and when someone will get their period. It's normal for menstrual cycles to vary from one person to another, but having very short, very long, or erratic cycles can signal fertility concerns.

This may all seem puzzling or even annoying, but I promise it all begins to make sense with proper tracking and awareness. By monitoring your cycle and identifying the signs we've discussed, you will gain key insights into your unique situation. With this knowledge in hand, you will transition from feeling confused and hopeless to having a clearer path forward to supporting your reproductive health. Here I discuss the most common conditions associated with irregular cycles, practical strategies to help you get back on track, and when to seek medical advice.

Polycystic Ovary Syndrome

Polycystic ovary syndrome (PCOS) is the most common hormonal condition in menstruating people. It's estimated that 5–15 percent of menstruating individuals have PCOS, and many are undiagnosed. PCOS is a major cause of infertility due to irregular ovulation and hormonal imbalances.

People with PCOS often experience a range of symptoms, including irregular periods, acne, excess facial hair, hair thinning on the scalp, elevated glucose levels, and weight gain. PCOS can also lead to other health issues, such as insulin resistance, high cholesterol, heart disease, obesity, diabetes, and depression.

PCOS wins the title of "most confusing name" because not everyone with PCOS has polycystic ovaries, and having polycystic ovaries (or ovarian cysts) doesn't mean you have PCOS!

Because PCOS is a syndrome, its symptoms can vary widely among individuals, making it challenging to identify or diagnose. It's important to note that not everyone with PCOS will exhibit all three criteria (outlined below); in fact, most individuals do not. Many people present with a combination of two of the listed criteria. If you're experiencing symptoms, especially if you've had fewer than eight periods in a year, discuss them with your healthcare provider to explore the possibility of PCOS.

Testing for PCOS

PCOS is diagnosed through a combination of medical history, physical examination, and specific tests. The widely accepted diagnostic criteria, known as the Rotterdam criteria, requires that individuals meet *two out of the following three* criteria.[1]

- Irregular, infrequent, or absent periods (occurring more than 35 days apart or less than eight times a year)

- High androgen levels detected on lab tests (such as elevated testosterone), or symptoms of high androgens, such as acne, facial hair, receding hairline, or thinning at the crown of the head

- Polycystic ovaries visible on ultrasound

Problems Associated with PCOS

On average, people with PCOS take longer to become pregnant. Infrequent, irregular, or missing periods mean that ovulation does not occur regularly. This can make timing intercourse difficult, and long cycles mean fewer opportunities to conceive.

Insulin resistance, the result of blood sugar imbalance, is a problem for 95 percent of overweight people with PCOS and 75 percent of lean people with PCOS.[2] Elevated androgens and increased testosterone can affect egg quality and contribute to insulin resistance. Chronic, low-grade inflammation is classically associated with PCOS and, as we've previously discussed, has a negative effect on overall health and fertility.

It is also important to know that PCOS is a chronic condition associated with long-term health issues including diabetes, high cholesterol, high blood pressure, and obesity. While your immediate goal may be a healthy baby, addressing the underlying imbalances specific to your PCOS presentation is crucial for your overall well-being in the long run.

The good news is that a PCOS diagnosis doesn't mean you won't be able to get pregnant. In fact, PCOS is considered one of the most common and treatable causes of infertility.

PREVALENCE OF DELAYED PCOS DIAGNOSIS: INSIGHTS FROM AN INTERNATIONAL STUDY

Researchers interviewed 1,385 people who had been diagnosed with PCOS to understand how they were diagnosed and what information they received about PCOS.[3] The results were surprising.

- Over a third (33.6 percent) of the people said it took more than 2 years to get a diagnosis.
- Almost half (47.1 percent) had to see three or more doctors before getting a diagnosis.
- Only 15.6 percent felt satisfied with the information they received.

If you're experiencing signs of PCOS or any health issue, don't be shy about seeking different opinions and pushing for the care and information you need.

Blood test results that are often associated with PCOS include:

- LH two to three times higher than FSH when tested on cycle day 3
- Elevated anti-Müllerian hormone (AMH)
- Elevated testosterone, DHT, DHEA-S
- Elevated fasting glucose, insulin, or HbA1c
- Elevated lipids

PCOS TERMINOLOGY

- **Secondary amenorrhea:** when a menstruating person does not get a period for 3 months or more

- **Oligomenorrhea:** infrequent menstrual periods (cycles are often more than 35 days with only six to eight periods a year)

- **Oligoovulation:** infrequent ovulation

- **Anovulation:** lack of ovulation

PCOS and Nutrition, Movement, Sleep, and Lifestyle Support

As far as treatment goes, it's possible to manage PCOS through nutrition, lifestyle changes, herbs, and supplements. This can help improve your chances of pregnancy and decrease your chances of long-term health issues. It is also possible to combine fertility treatments with certain recommendations (included below) for a holistic approach. The bottom line is that addressing PCOS doesn't end with getting pregnant and having a healthy baby. It's a long-term commitment to lowering your risk of associated health conditions.

NUTRITION

Dietary changes are the first, and often most important, strategy for addressing PCOS. Remember the nutrition pillars from Chapter 6: YES to nutrient-dense foods, YES to blood sugar balance, YES to gut health. Avoid trans fats, industrial seed oils, soda, and alcohol.

By following these guidelines, you'll be fueling your body in a way that supports balanced blood sugar, lowers the risk of insulin resistance, and reduces inflammation—all vital factors for managing PCOS.

Here are some key points to keep in mind that are particularly relevant for PCOS.

Don't eat carbs on their own. Always balance carbs with protein and healthy fats for better blood sugar balance.

Carbohydrate tolerance varies individually: Reducing carbohydrate intake can help with hormone balance, lower insulin, and improve ovulation, but restricting carbohydrates too much can have a negative effect on ovulation and fertility. The exact amount will vary for each person, but several studies have shown a benefit when carbs accounted for 30–40 percent of the diet.[4] For a 2,000-calorie diet, that would equate to 150–200 g of carbohydrates per day.

Protein is your friend for feeling full without spiking blood sugar. Aim for about 100 g daily. You may need more if you are more active.

Stick to regular meal times. Consistency supports your body's natural rhythms, including regular menstrual cycles and ovulation.

Avoid extremely low-fat, low-calorie, or very low-carb diets. These can trigger stress responses in the brain, potentially disrupting ovulation.

MOVEMENT

Exercise is incredibly important for managing PCOS because of the dramatic impact it can have on insulin resistance. Strengthening muscles through exercise enhances their ability to consume glucose, which helps to regulate blood sugar levels effectively. Additionally, exercise increases the sensitivity of muscle cells to insulin, reducing the need for excessive insulin production by the pancreas to maintain metabolic balance. Strength training can also help decrease androgen levels, particularly testosterone.

Cardiovascular exercise is also important. It burns fat and improves cardiovascular health. High-intensity interval training (HIIT) can be a particularly effective form of exercise for people with PCOS. Compared to moderate-intensity, continuous training (MICT), HIIT resulted in greater improvements in insulin sensitivity, menstrual cycle regularity, and reduction in hyperandrogenism in those with PCOS.[5]

Yoga also deserves a spot in your exercise repertoire. In addition to the general health benefits of yoga, a regular yoga practice can lower androgens in people with PCOS.

The goal is to be consistent, and make sure you are adequately fueling your body to support increased movement and muscle building. Try to incorporate some kind of movement every day. Think of it like a "menu of movement" and choose what is going to work best for you. Here are some ideas.

- A 20–30 minute HIIT workout, two or three times per week

- 30–45 minutes of strength training three to five times per week

- Walking, Pilates, or yoga on days you aren't doing HIIT, cardio, or strength training

Avoid overexercising and undereating! Pushing yourself to do an hour or more of strenuous exercise every day can have a negative impact on your stress hormones, which isn't good for your fertility or overall health.

Don't sacrifice adequate sleep to squeeze in workouts.

SLEEP AND CIRCADIAN RHYTHM

Getting enough sleep and sticking to a regular sleep routine is vital for individuals with PCOS, who often experience higher rates of sleep disturbances. Adequate sleep plays a role in balancing hormones related to the menstrual cycle, such as estrogen, progesterone, LH, and FSH. Disrupted sleep can also lead to or worsen insulin resistance, exacerbating symptoms of PCOS.

Additionally, disturbed sleep can throw off levels of leptin, a hormone that helps regulate body weight. Making sure you get good quality sleep is key to keeping these hormones in check and managing PCOS effectively.

Support your circadian rhythm and sleep cycle by reinforcing other daily cycles: going to sleep and waking around the same time every day, regular morning sunlight exposure, eating regular meals at predictable times, and regular times of activity. Gentle herbs (see Chapter 9 for specific herbs and recipes) as well as melatonin (see Supplements below) can also be used in the evening to help support the sleep cycle.

BPA AND OTHER ENDOCRINE-DISRUPTING CHEMICALS

As discussed in Chapter 10, BPA is a chemical used primarily in the production of polycarbonate plastics. Individuals with PCOS should pay particular attention to exposure to endocrine disruptors, particularly BPA. BPA has been linked to insulin resistance, polycystic ovaries, elevated testosterone levels, and low-grade chronic inflammation.[6] Refer to Chapter 10 for strategies to help reduce exposure.

Supplements to Assist with Fertility

Various supplements can assist with fertility in PCOS, but not all are necessary or beneficial for everyone. Matching your symptoms with the benefits seen in studies can help customize your supplement routine effectively.

INOSITOL

Inositol, a natural type of sugar found in the body and certain foods, is one of the most well-studied supplements for its benefits in PCOS. It can lower insulin, glucose, and testosterone levels; regulate ovulation; and possibly improve embryo quality.[7] In fact, studies showed inositol is as effective as metformin (a medication used to lower glucose levels) without the negative side effects. The myo-inositol form (versus the D-chiro-inositol form) is more helpful in PCOS, often combined in a 40:1 ratio.

Dosage ranges between 2 and 4 g per day, available in capsule or powder form. Powder mixes well in water or food and can be easier than taking the multiple capsules needed to reach 2–4 g daily.

VITAMIN D

Vitamin D deficiency is common in the general population but is found at even higher percentages in the PCOS population. It is one of the most important nutrients for people with PCOS. Supplementing with vitamin D can help with follicular development, menstrual cycle regulation, painful periods, lowering testosterone levels, improving insulin resistance, and decreasing inflammation.

Dosage is 1,000–4,000 IU per day. Test your vitamin D level first to better customize your supplementation dose and to maintain optimal levels.

OMEGA-3 FATTY ACIDS

Omega-3 fatty acids, found in fish oil, have many benefits for individuals with PCOS, most notably their ability to reduce inflammation. Supplementing with omega-3s can enhance ovulation and hormone production, promoting healthier egg development. Additionally, omega-3s may improve insulin resistance, lower triglycerides, and total cholesterol levels.

Dosage is 1.5–2 g of omega-3 fatty acids per day (choose a blend of DHA and EPA).

N-ACETYL-CYSTEINE (NAC)

NAC is an antioxidant that stimulates your own body's production of glutathione, one of the most important and potent antioxidants. Research has shown NAC can help improve metabolic disorders in individuals with PCOS. Taking NAC can lower blood sugar and cholesterol levels, and long-term use might even help with weight loss. Plus, studies show it can boost ovulation and pregnancy rates.[8] On top of that, it helps fight inflammation, which is important for managing PCOS symptoms.

Dosage is 1,500–1,800 mg per day.

MELATONIN

Melatonin, a hormone that helps regulate sleep–wake cycles and has strong antioxidant properties, shows promise in supporting PCOS by balancing sleep patterns and improving egg quality and ovulation while reducing androgens. PCOS appears to disrupt both the body's internal clock and melatonin levels, particularly ovarian melatonin levels. Research has shown significant hormone changes after 6 months of melatonin supplementation, including reductions in androgens, free testosterone, AMH, low-density lipoprotein, and improvement in menstrual regularity.[9] A study with melatonin and myo-inositol together improved oocyte and embryo quality and fertilization rates in IVF patients with PCOS.[10]

Dosage is 1–3 mg in the evening, 2–3 hours before going to bed.

Herbs to Address PCOS

Herbs play a role in addressing the underlying causes and symptoms of PCOS, such as insulin resistance, inflammation, irregular ovulation, and high androgen levels. For optimal results, it's essential to choose herbs that target your specific symptoms and to use them consistently over time.

BLOOD SUGAR AND INSULIN SUPPORT

Cinnamon bark. Cinnamon (*Cinnamomum* spp.) is one of the most commonly used spices in the world and has gained the attention of researchers for its ability to lower blood sugar and reduce insulin sensitivity. Additionally, studies have shown improved menstrual regularity,[11,12] a decrease in weight, and lower testosterone[13] in people with PCOS who take cinnamon. It's easy to get therapeutic doses by adding just ½–1 teaspoon of cinnamon to your food daily. Bonus: Sprinkling cinnamon on your food can also help reduce sugar cravings.

Use and dosage: 1–2 g of cinnamon per day, sprinkled over food or in beverages; ½ teaspoon equals approximately 1.5 g. Caution: If you tend to struggle with constipation, cinnamon may not be the herb for you. It is a classic remedy for diarrhea and can be constipating for some people.

Simple Cinnamon and Ginger Tea

I love the flavor combination of these two herbs, and together they help support PCOS in a synergistic way! One study compared the effects of cinnamon and ginger to the common medication metformin in people with PCOS. It found that 1.5 g of cinnamon per day decreased insulin resistance and testosterone levels while 1.5 mg of ginger significantly decreased FSH and LH levels.[14]

- 2   cinnamon sticks
- 1-2 teaspoons grated or chopped fresh ginger
- 1½   cups boiling water

Place the cinnamon, ginger, and boiling water in a pot and simmer, covered, for approximately 20 minutes. Strain and enjoy.

Alternatively, if you are on the go or don't want to take the time to simmer the tea on the stove, place the cinnamon and ginger in a thermos, cover with the boiling water, and let steep for at least 1 hour before drinking.

EXPLORING CINNAMON: NAVIGATING THE DIFFERENT TYPES

Ever wondered about the different types of cinnamon and if one is better than the other? It can be a bit confusing, especially with each type going by various, evolving Latin names over time!

Cinnamomum cassia is the most common cinnamon found in US grocery stores. It is also called Chinese cinnamon or cassia. It's the bold, spicy flavor you're likely familiar with in your spice cabinet.

Cinnamomum verum (formerly *C. zylanicum*) is known as "true" cinnamon, "sweet" cinnamon, or Ceylon cinnamon. This cinnamon is considered to be of superior quality to cassia, has a delicate and mildly sweet flavor, and is more expensive.

Coumarin is a compound found naturally in numerous plants, including cinnamon, that can be harmful in large doses. The amount naturally present in *C. cassia* is completely safe when used in small, culinary doses, but it theoretically poses a problem if you are taking higher doses over longer periods of time. The levels of coumarin in *C. verum* are so low that they are often undetectable.

Both cinnamons have been studied for health benefits, but *C. verum* shows the most promise and is what is often used with PCOS patients. It is also lower in coumarin, making this a safe choice when taking regularly in medicinal doses. It's not the variety commonly found in grocery stores, but natural food stores and high-quality online herbal stores will carry different types of cinnamon and clearly identify the variety on the packaging. Note: Always check the Latin name to verify which cinnamon you are purchasing.

HERBAL BITTERS

One of the most common hurdles my clients face is the relentless grip of sugar and carb cravings. It's a challenging cycle: The more sugar and carbs consumed, the stronger and more intense the signals from the brain to crave them. That's where herbal bitters step in to help break the cycle. Herbal bitters squash sugar cravings and help us feel full and satisfied without overeating. They are one of the best strategies for managing blood sugar and lipid imbalances, regulating appetite, and even reversing the metabolic syndrome. Bonus: Many people find bitters clear up acne and help their skin glow!

Dosage is 2–3 mL (about ½ teaspoon) of herbal bitter tincture in a small amount of water, 10–15 minutes before meals. Common herbs included in herbal bitters formulas include gentian, artichoke, dandelion root, chicory, burdock, ginger, and turmeric.

ANDROGEN SUPPORT

Symptoms of elevated androgen levels may include acne, facial hair, and receding or thinning hairline at the crown of the head.

Spearmint. Spearmint leaf (*Mentha spicata*) is one of the first teas I recommend to support clients with symptoms of elevated androgens, particularly unwanted facial hair and acne. Packed with antioxidants and anti-androgenic properties, spearmint tea works by helping to balance hormone levels, particularly testosterone, which can be elevated in individuals with PCOS. Studies showed that just 2 cups per day can help decrease testosterone levels and hirsutism (abnormal growth of hair on a person's face and body) in people with PCOS.[15]

Dosage is 2 cups of spearmint tea per day, approximately 2 g total (most tea bags contain 1 g of herb). Cover and steep for 10 minutes.

Peony and licorice. Peony (*Paeonia lactiflora*) root and licorice (*Glycyrrhiza glabra*) root are often combined for a synergistic approach to the complex hormonal imbalances in PCOS. The combination, a traditional Japanese formulation called Shakuyaku-kanzo-to, has been shown to lower testosterone, lower LH, improve ovulation, improve pregnancy rates,[16,17] and improve insulin response.[18]

Caution: Long-term use of high doses of licorice can increase blood pressure. Even short-term use is not suggested if you have hypertension. Deglycyrrhizinated licorice may be an alternative, but I recommend consulting your medical professional.

This combination is often found in tincture or capsule form; follow the directions on the label.

Reishi. This mushroom (*Ganoderma lucidum*) is highly regarded by herbalists for its ability to soothe the nervous system. In addition to its stress-relieving properties (see Chapter 9), reishi also deserves a place in the PCOS toolbox. It has been shown to lower androgen levels by inhibiting 5-alpha reductase, which is the enzyme that converts the inactive form of testosterone to its active form dihydrotestosterone (DHT), thereby decreasing DHT levels.[19] Reishi can also lower inflammation and help stabilize blood sugar levels—both crucial for PCOS management.

Reishi mushroom powder can be made as a tea or blended into warm beverages and coffees. Tinctures or capsules are also a convenient way to incorporate it into your day.

Dosage is 1–4 g (1 teaspoon equals about 3 g) per day of powder or 4–6 mL of tincture, two or three times per day. For capsules, follow the recommended dosage on the label.

OVULATION SUPPORT

Black cohosh. Black cohosh (*Actaea racemosa*) root is often recommended for a person with PCOS who has irregular, infrequent, or absent periods. Interestingly, Clomid (clomiphene) may work better and have fewer side effects when used in combination with black cohosh. One study compared a group of PCOS patients that was taking Clomid alone to a group that was taking Clomid with black cohosh. The black cohosh group had higher pregnancy rates, shorter cycles, lower LH, higher progesterone in the luteal phase,[20] and thicker uterine lining.[21]

Dosage is 2–4 mL, two or three times per day in tincture form. For capsule form, follow directions on the label.

Warning: Black cohosh is NOT safe in pregnancy. It is safe to take before and during ovulation, but stop 7–10 days after ovulating. Remember to always check the Herbs That Are Safe in Pregnancy list in Chapter 12 as soon as you know you are pregnant.

Vitex berry. Search "herbs for fertility," and vitex (*Vitex agnus-castus*) will usually be the top result. It's popular for good reason, helping with PMS symptoms, regulating ovulation, and boosting progesterone. However, it's not a cure-all solution for every fertility challenge and, in my view, is often overused. It's most effective when cycles are irregular or absent, as they often are in PCOS. Vitex works by stimulating dopamine activity, which lowers LH and prolactin, ultimately reducing testosterone and increasing progesterone.[22] This all helps improve ovulation and fertility.

Caution: Although most research finds vitex useful in PMS and hormone-related mood swings, some people find that it worsens low mood or depression. Always listen to your body.

Dosage is 500–1,000 mg per day in capsule form. Tincture form is 3–5 mL daily.

Cycle Tracking with PCOS

When you have PCOS and irregular cycles, figuring out the best time for intercourse can be a challenge. Ovulation may occur sporadically or not at all. Adding to the uncertainty, OPKs (ovulation predictor kits) are often unreliable for people with PCOS, giving false positives due to high LH levels throughout the month. But there are things you can do to help identify your fertile window and confirm ovulation.

Understanding how to track your cycle and time intercourse is crucial, especially with irregular or long cycles. The goal is to eventually establish regular ovulation using targeted herbs, supplements, and nutrition strategies for PCOS. However, in the meantime, you can still conceive with irregular cycles. The key is to recognize the signs that ovulation may be approaching.

Remember that your body produces estrogen as it's gearing up for ovulation, which prompts the cervix to produce cervical fluid. In PCOS, this process may start and stop multiple times over several weeks before ovulation actually occurs. Tracking cervical fluid and basal body temperature are essential clues.

Cervical fluid. Anytime you notice cervical fluid, you *may* be about to ovulate and are possibly fertile.

Basal body temperature. After ovulation, your temperature will rise and stay elevated, and your fertile window is closed for this cycle.

Any of the days that you notice cervical fluid, you are potentially in your fertile window. Having intercourse during these days increases your chances of pregnancy. It's common for this to happen multiple times in a PCOS cycle. You'll know ovulation has occurred, and your fertile window is over, when your basal body temperature rises and remains elevated for at least 3 days.

My client Lauren's experience charting is fairly typical of PCOS. She was diagnosed with PCOS by her doctor, and when we started working together, she struggled with irregular cycles and confusing OPK results. She would have a positive strip one day, then negative for a few days, then positive again for a few days. Her cycles ranged between 45 and 65 days long, and she was feeling frustrated about when to have intercourse. Tracking her cervical fluid was key to timing intercourse.

Once Lauren experienced cervical fluid on cycle days 20–22, 28–29, 34–36, and 41–44. On day 45, her temperature increased and remained elevated for 13 days until her period started, making the total cycle length 57 days. The elevated temperature on cycle day 45 confirmed ovulation on cycle day 44. As long as Lauren and her partner had intercourse anytime between day 41 and day 44, she would have a chance of pregnancy. Since you won't know if you ovulated until after the fact, having intercourse each time you notice cervical fluid will cover all the bases! Remember sperm can live for up to 5 days, so you don't need to have intercourse every day that you have cervical fluid (unless you want to). At least once for each cluster of cervical fluid days will suffice.

Armed with this information, when Lauren noticed cervical fluid on days 49–51, she and her partner had intercourse during this time frame. After noticing several clusters of cervical fluid, her temperature rose on day 52.

Remember that after 3 days of elevated temperature, Lauren could confirm ovulation had occurred. The moral of this story is that because Lauren noticed her cervical fluid, knew the indication of ovulation, and had sex, the likelihood of conception increased. Success! After 15 days of elevated temperature, and no period, Lauren took a pregnancy test and it was positive.

Remember, ovulation can happen at any time during your cycle. Lauren's story illustrates that conception is possible regardless of when it occurs. Trust the process and keep tracking!

Putting It All Together

PCOS is a lifelong condition that requires careful management. The steps involve obtaining an accurate diagnosis from your doctor, getting clear on your specific presentation of PCOS, and then building a personalized approach that supports your fertility and health goals. Whether prescription medications are included in your plan or not, your plan should encompass nutrition, lifestyle adjustments, and targeted supplements and herbs tailored to your particular constellation of symptoms and underlying causes. This comprehensive approach will support your fertility journey while also promoting long-term health and well-being.

Hypothalamic Amenorrhea

Hypothalamic amenorrhea (HA) is diagnosed when a person who previously had regular periods stops menstruating for 6 months or longer, after ruling out other medical causes. HA happens when there's a communication breakdown between the brain's hypothalamus and the ovaries, known as the HPO axis, so there is inadequate energy available, and this causes stress in the body.

In simple terms, the hypothalamus senses that something isn't right (not enough calories or nutrients to meet current energy demands) and decides it's not safe to have a baby. It slows down or stops sending out GnRH, which decreases FSH and LH. When FSH and LH levels drop, egg development slows or stops, and eventually the person with HA stops ovulating. No ovulation means no chance of pregnancy.

The three main causes of HA are undernutrition, overexercise, and stress. HA is often a combination of all three. Being nutrient deficient can occur from undereating, restricting nutrient-dense foods like healthy fats and proteins, or not eating enough for the level of activity. Contrary to popular belief, you don't have to be underweight to develop HA; it can affect those with normal BMIs as well. Genetics play a role, too, with some people more prone to losing their period at an energy-deficit level that another person may be able to tolerate. The bottom line is your menstrual cycle serves as a vital sign of overall health and fertility, and if it disappears, it must be addressed.

Typically, there are signs that show up months before a person completely loses their period. In the early stages of HA, signs include menstrual cycles shortening, spotting before the period begins, and/or little or no cervical fluid. Eventually, ovulation comes to a halt and the period stops altogether. This slow but steady regression can make diagnosing HA difficult.

Blood test results often associated with HA include:

- Normal to low FSH
- Normal to low LH
- Normal to low estradiol

- Normal to low TSH
- Normal AMH

IS IT PCOS OR HA?

While two very different conditions, PCOS and HA can potentially share clinical features, which can make getting a proper diagnosis tricky. Although PCOS and HA can exist alongside one another, it's more common for HA to go undiagnosed or be misdiagnosed. The strategies to address these two conditions are very different, so getting an accurate diagnosis matters.

WHERE PCOS AND HA CAN OVERLAP

POSSIBLE FINDINGS WITH PCOS	POSSIBLE FINDINGS WITH HA
Irregular or missing period: cycles are irregular or long–often 60 or more days without a period–but eventually, people with PCOS do get a period.	Irregular or missing period: the early stages of HA are typically irregular cycles, which then progress to no period.
Polycystic ovaries: found in about 75% of people with PCOS	Polycystic ovaries: found in about 30% of the general population

WHERE PCOS AND HA DIFFER

ASSOCIATED WITH PCOS	ASSOCIATED WITH HA
Elevated LH: often two to three times higher than FSH	Low to normal LH
Elevated androgens (testosterone, DHT, DHEA-S)	Normal androgens (testosterone, DHT, DHEA-S)
Normal FSH	Low to normal FSH
Normal to high estradiol	Low to normal estradiol
Normal to high TSH	Low to normal TSH
Elevated AMH	Normal AMH
Elevated glucose or insulin	Normal glucose or insulin
Thickened uterine lining	Thin to normal uterine lining

The good news is that since HA is not a disorder but is rather the body's natural response to perceiving an unsafe environment for pregnancy, it is completely reversible. Addressing the root cause is critical to kick-starting your menstrual cycle and getting you back on the fertile track.

Supporting nutrition and decreasing stress—both physical stress and psychological stress—is foundational for recovery and key for getting your body ovulating again. Once the underlying cause of your HA has been identified, herbs can support your road to fertility. With a combined, comprehensive approach, many people start ovulating and get their period back in 2–3 months. (It may take longer, which is often correlated with how long the period has been absent.)

What does this all-encompassing approach look like? It's a combination of the energy balance between food, activity, and stress levels. And yes, if you have an HA diagnosis, all of these need to be addressed.

Nutrition

When it comes to addressing the HA energy balance through diet, it's not just about consuming more calories. The key is to ensure you're getting enough nutrient-rich protein, healthy fats, and carbohydrates. The strategies in Chapter 6 are a good place to start, but here are a few tips specific to HA.

Include all three macronutrients at every meal. That means protein, fat, and carbohydrates. Now is not the time to go low-carb, low-fat, or low-cal!

Skip intermittent fasting (IF). While very popular in the fitness community, IF sends a stress signal to your brain in response to low glucose levels, which lowers the hormones needed for egg development and ovulation. It's also hard to hit calorie and nutrient goals if you are eating within a shorter window of time. Instead, eat within 1 hour of waking and don't skip meals.

Listen to your hunger cues. If you feel hungry within an hour or two of eating, you may need more protein to stay full longer. Snack when you are hungry, making sure each snack contains protein, carbohydrates, and fat.

Everything is fine in moderation. If you find yourself holding on to the belief that there are "bad" foods and "good" foods, here's your gentle reminder that all foods are okay in moderation. Should you get all of your calories from burgers, fries, fancy lattes, pizza, and ice cream? No. But having these foods occasionally is absolutely okay!

If any of these recommendations feel scary, overwhelming, or triggering, consider working with a professional trained in disordered eating. Nutritionists, registered dietitians, and therapists can help you work through any challenges that may be getting in the way of a healthy relationship between yourself and food.

Movement

Daily movement is an important part of a healthy lifestyle and fertility plan. However, it's all about balance! The sweet spot lies in making sure your total activity level isn't too much of a stress on your body and that you are fueling enough to meet the energy demands. Here are some guidelines.

Limit to 1 hour daily. Keep your exercise and strenuous activities to no more than 1 hour per day.

Take rest days. Let your body rest 1–2 days per week. Depending on how long it's been since you had a period and how significant the energy imbalance is, you may need to rest more.

Use the "talk test." You should be able to talk while exercising and not feel exhausted or depleted after exercising.

Sleep

Getting a good night's sleep is an important part of managing stress and supporting hormones. Chapter 9 covers sleep more broadly, but here are some points to consider in the context of HA.

Get enough. Aim for a minimum of 7 hours of sleep per night, preferably 8–9 hours.

Prioritize sleep. While recovering from HA, it is critical that your body has plenty of time to rest. If the choice is between another hour of sleep or waking to squeeze in a workout, choose sleep.

Stick to a routine. Going to bed and waking at approximately the same time every day helps support your circadian rhythm, which helps regulate reproductive and stress hormones.

Sleep in complete darkness. Use blackout shades, curtains, or an eye mask to keep all light out of the bedroom. Even relatively dim light—equivalent to a hallway light—can prevent you from entering deep sleep, thus having a negative effect on reproductive hormones.

Herbs for HA

Herbs are a potent ally in the recovery from HA, but remember, they're just one piece of the puzzle. You can't skip working on the root causes and think that herbs will get you a healthy ovulation and period. Here are some of my go-to herbs when supporting patients with HA.

A strong herbal infusion is nutritious and nourishing and just what the body is craving as it's recovering from HA. Herbs such as nettle leaf, oat straw, and red clover (*Trifolium pratense*) provide a large dose of vitamins and minerals, particularly calcium, magnesium, and iron.

Overnight Infusion for HA

¼ cup dried nettle leaf

¼ cup dried oat straw

¼ cup dried red clover

32 ounces (4 cups) boiling water

Place the herbs in a 32-ounce glass jar with a lid or in a large French press. Fill with the boiling water. Put the lid on and let steep for at least 4 hours or overnight. Use a mesh strainer or the French press to strain out the herbs. Drink 2 cups per day at the temperature you prefer. Store leftover infusion in the refrigerator and drink within 24 hours.

Time-saver tip: To make a large batch of this herbal mixture at once, mix all the herbs together and store in an airtight container in a cool, dark place. Scoop out about ¾ cup of the mixture when making your overnight infusion.

MACA ROOT

Maca (*Lepidium meyenii*) is a nutritive herb rich in essential amino acids, iodine, iron, and magnesium. Its high-nutrient content and ability to increase FSH and LH make maca a supportive ally for people with HA.

Maca powder can be mixed into smoothies, coffee, or other foods. The Maca Nut Butter Balls recipe in Chapter 8 is a delicious snack to help meet your nutrient needs.

Typical Dosage Ranges

Powder: 2–8 g (1 teaspoon equals about 4 g) per day
Tincture: 4–6 mL, two or three times per day
Capsules: Follow the recommended dosage on the label

SHATAVARI

Shatavari (*Asparagus racemosus*) root is a renowned Ayurvedic herb, celebrated for its rejuvenating properties that enhance vitality and overall health. With a rich tradition of use, it has been cherished for its ability to improve fertility, hormone balance, and lactation. As an adaptogen, shatavari aids the body's response to stress, while its antistress and antioxidant qualities are especially beneficial in cases of HA, nurturing the HPO axis and ovulation.

Typical Dosage Ranges

Tea: 1–2 tablespoons of dried shatavari root, simmered over the stove for 20 minutes
Powder: Between 2 and 10 g per day (start low and work your way up, stopping if it bothers your stomach)
Tincture: 5–15 mL per day
Capsules: Follow the recommended dosage on the label

Shatavari Hot Chocolate

1 cup full-fat coconut milk
1 tablespoon honey
1 tablespoon raw cacao powder
½ teaspoon shatavari root powder
¼ teaspoon pure vanilla extract
Pinch of salt

Combine all the ingredients in a pot and gently heat until hot, but not boiling. Enjoy hot.

VITEX

Vitex berry, also known as chaste tree berry, is one of the most popular "fertility herbs." However, its widespread promotion online has led many people to misuse it for fertility issues it may not effectively address. There are many factors that contribute to a person having difficulty conceiving, and while vitex can be helpful for certain aspects of fertility challenges, it's not a one-size-fits-all solution (no herb is!).

Where vitex shines is in its ability to help support the communication between the pituitary gland and the ovaries to help restore ovulation and menstruation. Vitex encourages the pituitary gland to increase LH production, which in turn supports ovulation and the formation of the corpus luteum. This process is crucial for maintaining healthy progesterone levels during the latter part of the menstrual cycle.

Caution: Some people find that vitex worsens low mood or depression. Always listen to your body.

Typical Dosage Ranges

Tincture: 3–5 mL per day
Capsules: 500–1,000 mg per day

REISHI AND ELEUTHERO ROOT

Introduced in Chapter 9 as stress reducers, both of these are particularly supportive for overcoming HA. Reishi is my go-to for anyone who is feeling anxious, moody, stressed, or having trouble sleeping—particularly when their dreams are waking them up. Eleuthero is helpful for those who feel burnt out, overworked, exhausted or stressed or have perfectionistic tendencies. It has historically been used to help people recovering from anorexia get their periods back, likely due to its effect on the stress response system and the HPO axis. I often combine reishi and eleuthero into a formula for my HA clients. Refer to Chapter 9 for more information.

Typical Dosage Ranges

Tea: 1–2 teaspoons of dried herb in 10–12 ounces of boiling water, 1–3 cups per day
Powder: 2–3 g (1 teaspoon equals about 2.5 g) per day
Tincture: 4–6 mL, two or three times per day
Capsules: Follow the recommended dosage on the label

MEGAN'S STORY
Overcoming HA

When Megan and her partner were ready to have a baby, they knew they would need help. As a same-sex couple, they had already selected their sperm donor and decided that Megan would provide the egg and carry the pregnancy. The problem was that over the last year, Megan's cycle had started to become irregular. What was once a consistent 30-day cycle had transitioned to irregular shorter cycles for a few months, and then stopped altogether. After ruling out other causes, her doctor diagnosed her with HA. The "prescription" was to eat more, exercise less, and gain weight. Megan was shocked by this diagnosis. She hadn't been intentionally dieting and her weight was basically the same as it had been for most of her adult life. How could this be?

When we dug deeper into her life over the past year, it all became clear. Megan was in a high-pressure job as a lawyer. Exercise was how she managed her stress; early-morning spin classes, runs with her partner before dinner, and often long bike rides or hikes on the weekend. She was conscious of "eating healthy," but sometimes her schedule didn't allow time for a big meal so she'd reach for a quick protein smoothie or bar. A seemingly healthy lifestyle, right?

Although Megan wasn't deliberately restricting her food intake, she wasn't consuming enough nutrients or calories to adequately fuel all of her activities. Additionally, she was under a lot of work stress, which can trigger hormonal changes. Altogether, Megan's brain was getting a clear message—not enough resources to reproduce.

MEGAN'S PROTOCOL

Movement. Limit exercise to 1 hour, three times per week. Short walks, stretching, or yoga on nonexercise days. Hiking or biking on weekends, but use the "talk test" to stay in a healthy range.

Nutrition. No skipping meals! Eat breakfast within an hour of waking, and focus on whole foods. Leave the protein bars for part of a balanced snack.

Sleep. Prioritize 8–9 hours per night. No waking early for workouts.

Herbs. Eleuthero tincture to help support her work stress, Maca Nut Butter Balls for nutrients and an easy snack, and Golden Milk with ¼ teaspoon of shatavari in the evening to help unwind.

Four months after making these changes and integrating herbs into her routine, Megan's period returned. After 6 months of regular periods, she and her partner felt ready to try to get pregnant and had success with their second IUI!

Remember that HA is not a disease; it's your body's way of letting you know it needs more nourishment, rest, stress support, and/or sleep. It's a completely reversible state. When you are trying to conceive, it's essential to begin from a state of abundance, ensuring you have the resources to sustain both your own well-being and the needs of a developing baby.

Premature Ovarian Insufficiency

Premature ovarian insufficiency (POI), previously known as premature menopause or premature ovarian failure, happens when the ovaries stop working as they should *before* age 40. POI affects about 1 percent of people. It is characterized by a lack of menstruation for at least 4 months combined with high FSH and low estradiol. Typically, a person experiences a gradual decline in menstrual frequency, with cycles becoming shortened, prolonged, or irregular before completely stopping. Some people experience symptoms similar to those in menopause, like hot flashes, night sweats, and vaginal dryness. POI is not the same as early menopause in that POI is not always permanent and intermittent ovulation may still occur, especially in the early stage of the condition.

There is not a lot known about POI and what causes it. Initial research shows that it may be linked to genetics, autoimmune diseases, infections, environmental factors, or medical treatments like chemotherapy.

Blood test results often associated with POI include:

- High FSH, greater than 25 IU/L on two occasions, more than 4 weeks apart

- Low estradiol

- Low AMH

What does this mean for your fertility? When the ovaries stop functioning normally, ovulation can be erratic or stop completely, making conception very difficult. It's not impossible, however, and between 5 and 10 percent of women with POI still conceive, as the function of the ovaries can fluctuate.[23] Pregnancies can occur naturally, with hormone replacement therapy, or through IVF, but often, egg donation is the only solution.

If you have a diagnosis of POI, it is important to meet with a reproductive endocrinologist to understand your options. Time is of the essence, as your chances of success with your own eggs are greater if you are under 35 years old.

In addition to meeting with a fertility doctor to understand all of your options, there are things you can do to help improve your chances of being one of the 5–10 percent of cases resulting in pregnancy with your own eggs. Following the recommendations in this book is a great starting point and will help support your health and fertility with an emphasis on egg quality. As an added bonus, you will also be optimizing the quality of your partner's sperm.

Adaptogen Herbs to Address POI

Adaptogen herbs help mitigate the effects of stress on the body. POI can be a stressful condition, both physically and emotionally, and chronic stress can exacerbate hormonal imbalances and other symptoms associated with POI. Adaptogens also help overall well-being and resilience, which can be beneficial as you navigate the challenges of POI and your fertility journey. While adaptogens may not directly address the underlying root cause of POI, they may complement other treatment approaches by promoting a sense of calm, supporting energy levels, and enhancing overall health and vitality.

The following adaptogens previously covered are worth considering: eleuthero, reishi, ashwagandha, shatavari, and schisandra berry.

Luteal Phase Deficiency

As a reminder, the luteal phase begins after ovulation and continues until the start of your next period. The average luteal phase lasts for 14 days, but can range from 12 to 16 days.

During the luteal phase, the corpus luteum—which is created when the empty follicle transforms after ovulation—secretes the hormone progesterone, needed to maintain an early pregnancy. This rise in progesterone causes the endometrial lining of the uterus to thicken, making it receptive to implantation of an embryo. As the luteal phase ends, progesterone levels begin to fall, which triggers menstruation. If the luteal phase is too short, an embryo may not have enough time to implant before flow begins.

In luteal phase deficiency (LPD), the corpus luteum starts to break down earlier than is typical. LPD is characterized by low progesterone and a luteal phase of 10 days or less.

Blood test results associated with LPD often include low progesterone—less than 10 ng/mL, when tested 7 days after confirmed ovulation.

While the exact cause of LPD is unclear, the following factors could be at play: undereating, nutrient deficiencies, overexercising, stress, illness, hyperprolactinemia, thyroid disorders, and PCOS.

Treating LPD often involves supplementing with progesterone during the luteal phase of the menstrual cycle. However, this approach may not address the underlying cause. If the ovaries struggle to produce enough progesterone for at least 10 days following ovulation (ideally enough for 12–14 days), it suggests they may need more comprehensive support. Understanding why the corpus luteum isn't functioning optimally will help address the root problem. Taking a holistic approach by supporting the entire menstrual cycle, rather than just relying on progesterone supplementation, offers a more comprehensive solution.

Strategies to Address LPD

There are several strategies for addressing LPD that involve supporting the entire cycle with a root cause approach.

REINFORCE DAILY RHYTHMS

Have you ever traveled across time zones and noticed your period was a few days late or early that month? Our circadian rhythm can influence the menstrual cycle, so creating regular daily rhythms is foundational to a healthy, regular period. Here are some strategies.

- Go to sleep and wake at the same time every day.

- Eat meals at the same time every day.

- Get 10–20 minutes of sunlight in the morning to increase melatonin levels that evening.

- Sleep in a completely dark room or wear an eye mask.

NUTRITION

I can't stress this enough—adequate nutrition is essential for healthy follicular development and egg maturation. A healthy follicle turns into a healthy corpus luteum after ovulation, which produces healthy levels of progesterone. Fueling your body for fertility, as outlined in Chapter 6, is the foundation for supporting LPD.

STRESS MANAGEMENT

Stress affects the HPO axis and can play a role in LPD. Stress and stress hormones (like cortisol) signal to the brain that it's not an ideal time to reproduce, and in response, the hypothalamus decreases the frequency or the speed of GnRH pulsation, which kicks off a domino effect resulting in lower estrogen, decreased LH surge, weaker corpus luteum, and ultimately lower progesterone.

Often LPD develops before a person progresses into hypothalamic amenorrhea, so managing stress can help catch issues earlier.

HORMONE SUPPORT

The following adaptogens and adaptogen-like herbs previously covered can be helpful for addressing LPD: eleuthero, reishi, ashwagandha, maca, shatavari, and schisandra berry. (See Chapter 9 for more information and yummy recipes.)

VITEX BERRY

Vitex, as previously discussed, helps support the communication between the pituitary gland and the ovaries to help regulate ovulation and support healthy progesterone levels. A popular recommendation is to take vitex only in the luteal phase to support progesterone, but in reality, vitex works best when taken regularly for the entire cycle, and this schedule is easier to remember, too! Remember, a healthy follicle turns into a healthy corpus luteum, and taking vitex in the beginning of your cycle helps support this process. Studies have shown vitex can address LPD by increasing cycle length, increasing progesterone levels, and increasing pregnancy rates.[24]

Caution: Some people find that vitex worsens low mood or depression. Always listen to your body.

Typical Dosage Ranges

Tincture: 3–5 mL per day
Capsules: 500–1,000 mg per day

MAGNESIUM

Often referred to as the "relaxation mineral," magnesium has a huge role to play in regulating hormones. Progesterone, estrogen, and testosterone are all created with the help of magnesium, so having sufficient levels can help with optimal hormone production and healthy progesterone levels. Magnesium can also be calming, decrease stress, and support restful sleep.

Common reasons for insufficient magnesium levels include a lack of magnesium-rich foods, foods that contain less magnesium as a result of declining soil quality, and stress.

Typical Dosage Ranges

Capsules: 100–300 mg capsules per day of magnesium glycinate or bisglycinate

Endometriosis

Endometriosis (also called endo) is a condition where tissue, similar to the lining of the uterus, grows in places it shouldn't. These bits of tissue, called endometrial lesions, can pop up in different spots but are often found in the abdominal cavity, around the uterus, ovaries, and fallopian tubes. Sometimes they show up in places like the bowel, bladder, or even the lungs.

Just as the lining of your uterus thickens and sheds, triggered by hormonal changes, these endometrial lesions do the same, causing them to bleed when you get your period. This bleeding outside of the uterus leads to pain and inflammation. Ten percent or more of menstruating people have endometriosis, and 30–40 percent of these people will experience fertility problems.

Getting a diagnosis of endometriosis can be tricky, often taking several years and multiple doctors. While the most common symptom of endometriosis is debilitating menstrual cramps—the kind of pain that leaves you doubled over in agony, or curled up on the bathroom floor, vomiting—this pain is not always consistent in intensity and location, and in some cases, is nonexistent. To complicate matters further, neither the quantity nor the severity of endometrial lesions seem to be linked to the level of pain a person feels. Endometriosis typically progresses with time, with chronic inflammation resulting in the buildup of scar tissue and the formation of adhesions. These adhesions can anchor organs in position, resulting in persistent pain, increased pain with bowel movements and urination, and painful sex.

What Causes It

There are multiple theories around the cause of and contributing factors to developing endometriosis, but the biggest driver appears to be inflammation and immune dysregulation. Endometrial lesions trigger the immune system to kick into gear in an attempt to rid the body of this misplaced tissue. If the immune system struggles in this process, a state of long-term inflammation ensues. New evidence points to the health of the intestinal bacteria playing a critical role in the development and progression of endometriosis.[25]

Endometrial lesions are also influenced by hormonal changes and worsened by exposure to endocrine-disrupting chemicals in our environment. While endometriosis is often viewed as a hormonal condition related to excess estrogen, the reality is more complex. Simply reducing estrogen levels, often done by prescribing birth control pills, does not address the underlying areas of immune dysfunction and inflammation.

So how does all of this relate to your road to pregnancy? Simply put, endo makes it harder to get pregnant. All of the side effects tell us why.

- Inflammation affects the quality of eggs and the ability of an embryo to attach to the uterus.

- Sperm don't swim well in an inflamed environment and can have trouble binding to the egg.

- Lesions on the ovaries can upset ovarian function.

- Scar tissue in the fallopian tubes or uterus makes it tougher for fertilization and implantation to happen.

Treatments for endometriosis usually rely on pain medications, surgery to remove lesions, or hormonal therapies, such as birth control pills. Surgery can clear the lesions, but they often come back. Birth control pills help manage the pain, but they don't get to the main drivers of inflammation and immune dysregulation and are obviously not an option when you are trying to get pregnant.

A holistic approach to endometriosis can greatly reduce painful symptoms and the inflammation that is causing the progression of endometriosis, ultimately affecting your fertility. I have seen firsthand how these changes can dramatically reduce a person's pain and help them get pregnant. However, addressing endometriosis takes time and a multifaceted approach, which may include working with an experienced surgeon to remove lesions or a fertility doctor if tubal scarring or ovarian function is an issue. Combining the strategies here with the guidance of a skilled healthcare team will give you your best chance of pregnancy. Below are the specific areas where lifestyle changes combined with an herbal plan will help.

Addressing the Pain

This is the first step! You simply cannot make lasting changes in other areas of your life if you're dealing with significant pain. The following herbs top my list for helping reduce painful periods, whether associated with endometriosis or not. The key to pain management is to stay ahead of the pain, meaning you start a pain protocol at the very first sign of pain, or before, if possible.

Ginger. Ginger (*Zingiber officinale*) is the first herb I reach for to help with period pain. Multiple studies have shown ginger decreases the severity and duration of pain, with some even showing it to be as effective as ibuprofen, without the possible side effects.[26] Quite the opposite to over-the-counter pain meds, ginger supports digestion and the microbiome, both of which can be disrupted with endometriosis. Ginger is a strong anti-inflammatory herb that inhibits prostaglandins—the chemicals in the body that trigger menstrual uterine contraction and pain.

The typical dosage of 2 g per day is found to be most effective for managing pain. It is safe to go higher as long as you know you are not pregnant. Take as early as possible and continue until the pain has passed.

Ginger can be taken in the form of capsules (500 mg, four times per day) or tea, such as the Lemon Ginger Tea from Chapter 8.

Cramp bark. Known for its ability to ease uterine cramping and muscle spasms, tincture of cramp bark (*Viburnum opulus*) can work fast and reliably. I find it particularly helpful for the type of period pain that radiates around the back and down the thighs. Similar to ginger and other allies in pain management, it is most effective when taken at the earliest onset of discomfort. Having a small bottle within reach, whether in your bag or on your nightstand, offers fast access to this herb when needed.

Typical dosage is 1 mL of tincture in a small amount of water at the first sign of pain. Repeat dose every 15 minutes until pain subsides, not to exceed 15 mL per day. Preventatively, take 5 mL (1 teaspoon) daily for a few days before the expected period.

Magnesium. This essential mineral plays a crucial role in muscle relaxation and pain relief, making it a go-to natural remedy for easing period cramps and uterine spasms. Similar to ginger, magnesium decreases prostaglandin levels, which leads to a decrease in menstrual cramps. Magnesium deficiency can also trigger the release of inflammatory molecules, exacerbating inflammation, which is already an issue with endometriosis.

Typical dosage is capsules of magnesium glycinate or bisglycinate, 100–400 mg per day.

Addressing Diet

The goal of an endo-focused diet is to decrease inflammation, increase natural detoxification, support gut health, and possibly eliminate gluten.

Inflammation. Anti-inflammatory foods help minimize the chronic inflammation that is driving endometriosis growth, progression, and symptoms. Try incorporating more foods like fruits, vegetables, whole grains, fatty fish, legumes, nuts, and seeds and avoid foods that contain high levels of added sugar, starches that are quickly converted into sugar (like white bread), and all highly processed foods, including packaged snacks and fried foods. Herbal tip: Green tea and turmeric are powerful anti-inflammatory allies! Check out the recipes in Chapter 8 for my favorite green tea or golden milk with turmeric.

Natural detoxification. Endometrial lesions are sensitive to estrogen, so helping the body clear out excess estrogen efficiently is beneficial. Eating cruciferous vegetables is one of the best ways to help your liver with gentle, daily detoxification. Cruciferous vegetables are unique because they're rich in glucosinolates, sulfur-containing compounds that aid in the body's detoxification process. Incorporate several servings of the following veggies every day: cauliflower, cabbage, kale, collard greens, bok choy, broccoli, Brussels sprouts, and arugula. Herbal tip: A daily cup of dandelion root tea or a tincture of digestive bitters can help give your liver a little extra support to naturally detoxify estrogen, medications, and other metabolic waste.

Microbiome. When the microbiome is out of balance, this contributes to more inflammation, and people with endometriosis often have more problematic bacteria in the gut. Follow the recommendations in Chapter 6 to shift your microbiome toward a healthier balance, and consider taking a probiotic supplement.

Gluten. Many people find that cutting out gluten helps with their endometriosis symptoms. One study showed a significant improvement in symptoms in 75 percent of the 207 people in the study after ditching gluten.[27] I've found that cutting out gluten appears to be particularly beneficial for individuals with endometriosis who also experience gastrointestinal issues such as gas, pain, and bloating.

Reducing Inflammation

Inflammation is a consistent and significant factor in endometriosis, and managing it is a big part of a holistic strategy. While much can be done through diet, there are additional supplements to consider, along with the herbs already mentioned (ginger, turmeric, and green tea).

N-acetyl-cysteine (NAC). NAC is an antioxidant that stimulates your own body's production of glutathione, one of the most important and potent antioxidants. NAC downregulates inflammation, and studies have shown it can decrease the size of endometrial lesions and reduce pain.[28]

Typical dosage is 1,500–1,800 mg per day.

Omega-3 fatty acids. Found in supplements like fish oil, omega-3 fatty acids are one of the most studied supplements on endometriosis. Research suggests omega-3 supplementation could slow the growth of endometrial lesions and reduce pain. Additionally, higher levels of EPA, a type of omega-3 fatty acid, is linked to a lower likelihood of having endometriosis altogether.[29]

Typical dosage is 1.5–2 g of omega-3 fatty acids per day (blend of DHA and EPA).

Decrease exposure to endocrine-disrupting chemicals (EDCs): Endometrial lesions have higher estrogen levels and don't handle estrogen as well as other tissues do. This means that decreasing exposure to chemicals that act like estrogen in the body (known as EDCs) can be helpful. Simple steps, like opting for organic products, using fewer plastic containers, avoiding cans lined with BPA, and steering clear of artificial fragrances, can make a significant difference. For more tips on how to reduce exposure to EDCs, check out Chapter 10.

Endometriosis is a lifelong condition and a journey that can be difficult and frustrating to manage. To see success, it's all about committing to a mix of strategies and keeping an open mind about what works best for you. By collaborating with your healthcare team and incorporating the natural strategies discussed here, you're giving yourself the best shot at managing the ups and downs of this condition and reclaiming some control over your life and fertility.

Ginger, Turmeric, and Lemon Balm Tea

This blend combines the anti-inflammatory power of ginger and turmeric.

1	tablespoon dried lemon balm
½	teaspoon ground turmeric
½	teaspoon ground ginger
8	ounces boiling water
	Juice from ¼–½ lemon

Combine the lemon balm, turmeric, and ginger in a mesh tea basket in a mug. Add the boiling water and lemon juice. Cover and steep for 10 to 15 minutes. Remove the tea basket and enjoy.

DANIELLE AND HANNAH'S STORIES
Addressing Endometriosis

DANIELLE'S STORY

When Danielle was a teenager, her periods were agonizing, causing her to miss out on school, family gatherings, and fun with friends. Over-the-counter pain meds barely made a dent. At 16, her doctor suggested birth control pills to help manage her cycle and pain, and they did the trick. Fast-forward 15 years, and Danielle was eager to start a family and stopped taking the pill. Pain and heavy bleeding returned with a vengeance. Her doctor suspected endometriosis, but the only way to confirm it was through laparoscopic surgery. Danielle decided to hold off on surgery and focused on getting pregnant. That's when I met her.

Our first step was to tackle the pain. Danielle started drinking ginger tea and reaching for cramp bark tincture at the first sign of discomfort, along with taking magnesium throughout the month. We also devised a plan to reduce her exposure to hormone-disrupting chemicals by cutting back on plastics, cleaning up her beauty routine, and filtering her tap water.

For diet, she added lots of anti-inflammatory foods, reduced processed foods, added four servings of cruciferous veggies daily, and sipped dandelion root tea to help her body metabolize and eliminate excess estrogen. On top of this, she took a mix of supplements, including a prenatal multivitamin, fish oil, probiotic, vitamin D, and NAC. Danielle kept a symptoms journal to track her pain, ovulation signs, and menstrual cycle.

After 2 months, she noticed a 20 percent reduction in pain, and by 5 months, it was cut in half. She got pregnant in her sixth month of tracking.

While Danielle achieved her goal of a healthy pregnancy, her journey with endometriosis didn't end there. After giving birth, she continued using natural strategies to manage symptoms and address the biggest drivers of endometriosis while working with her healthcare team to explore medical options if necessary.

HANNAH'S STORY

Another client, Hannah, faced similar challenges with endometriosis, but her journey and family planning strategy took a different turn. Like Danielle, Hannah battled excruciating periods during her teenage years, but when she tried oral contraceptives, her body didn't react well. She experienced a host of side effects, including weight gain and depression, ultimately deciding the pill wasn't for her. Throughout her 20s, she relied heavily on over-the-counter pain relievers.

At 29, after a year of unsuccessful attempts to conceive, Hannah sought my help. Mirroring Danielle's experience, Hannah began to notice a decrease in pain after only a few months of working together. However, she also struggled with digestive issues—gas, pain, bloating, and alternating constipation and diarrhea—prompting her to adopt a gluten-free diet, which brought relief to her GI symptoms and continued improvement in period pain. After 6 months, her pain decreased by about 40 percent, but still no pregnancy.

Suspecting endometriosis, Hannah's gynecologist recommended a laparoscopic surgery to investigate further. The procedure revealed significant endometrial lesions around her uterus, fallopian tubes, and one ovary. The surgeon removed as much as possible without compromising her ovary. Following recovery, Hannah consulted a reproductive endocrinologist, who advised that IVF offered her the best chance of conceiving. The inflammation and potential scarring from the lesions near her reproductive organs could impact various stages of the conception process. Throughout her IVF journey, Hannah used the strategies in this book to support her overall fertility, digestive health, and endometriosis symptoms. After her second IVF cycle, she successfully became pregnant and welcomed a healthy baby into the world.

Fibroids

Fibroids are noncancerous growths in the muscle of the uterus and are quite common. It's estimated that over 70 percent of individuals with a uterus will develop fibroids by the age of 50. The majority of fibroids cause little or no symptoms, with about 30 percent of people experiencing unpleasant symptoms such as heavy bleeding, feeling of fullness in the lower abdomen, cramping, bleeding between periods, pain during sex, frequent urination, constipation, or bloating. Fibroids grow an average of 20–30 percent in size per year until menopause, when the growth will typically stop.

The good news is that fibroids don't typically get in the way of getting pregnant or having a healthy pregnancy. In a small number of cases, depending on the size and location, fibroids might affect fertility by blocking the fallopian tubes, changing the shape of the uterus, or making it difficult for a fertilized egg to implant properly. Heavy bleeding often associated with fibroids can lead to anemia, which can also affect fertility.

If you suspect you have fibroids, it is important to work with your doctor for a thorough evaluation. Treatment, including surgery, may be necessary in the rare case that your fibroids are affecting your ability to get pregnant or your symptoms are severe. Whether or not medical treatment is necessary, natural approaches can be helpful in addressing symptoms and slowing fibroid growth.

Diet

Studies suggest that a higher intake of fruits, especially citrus fruits, and vegetables is linked to a reduced risk of fibroids. Conversely, alcohol consumption, particularly beer, may increase the risk of developing fibroids. Follow the guidelines in Chapter 6 to fuel your fertility, with a specific goal of 8–10 servings of fruits and veggies per day, with 1 serving of citrus fruits, and at least 3 servings of cruciferous veggies (cauliflower, cabbage, kale, collard greens, bok choy, broccoli, Brussels sprouts, arugula).

Lifestyle

While systemic blood levels of estrogen and progesterone are typically normal, uterine fibroid tissue often has elevated levels of these hormones. Reduce exposure to environmental endocrine-disrupting chemicals (EDCs) so that you are not adding to the increased levels of hormones at localized fibroid level. For tips on how to reduce exposure to EDCs, check out Chapter 10.

Supplements

Vitamin D. Vitamin D deficiency is associated with an increased risk of fibroids, and studies have shown that vitamin D supplementation can slow or halt fibroid progression. Optimal vitamin D levels are typically achieved with supplementation ranging from 2,000 to 4,000 IU, though individual needs may vary. It's essential to get tested to determine your precise levels and consult a healthcare professional to maintain optimal levels. Avoid exceeding 4,000 IU daily without medical supervision, and account for all supplement sources.

Iron. Screen for iron deficiency if menstrual bleeding is heavy and supplement as necessary.

Herbs

Green tea. An extract of green tea, EGCG, taken in capsule form, has been shown to decrease fibroid size and symptoms.

Typical dosage: While taking high levels of EGCG is not recommended when trying to conceive, drinking 1–3 cups of green tea daily is safe and may help slow fibroid growth.

Cinnamon. Beyond being a delicious spice, cinnamon (*Cinnamomum* spp.) has shown promise in reducing the heavy menstrual bleeding and pain associated with fibroids.

Typical dosage is 1–2 g of cinnamon per day, sprinkled over food or in beverages (½ teaspoon equals approximately 1.5 g). Caution: If you tend to struggle with constipation, cinnamon may not be the herb for you. It is a classic remedy for diarrhea and can be constipating for some people.

Ginger Cinnamon Tea

In this twist on the Lemon Ginger Tea from Chapter 8, the addition of cinnamon can help decrease heavy menstrual bleeding, while ginger helps decrease cramping.

1-2 teaspoons grated or chopped fresh ginger (no need to peel)

1 cinnamon stick or ½ teaspoon ground cinnamon

8 ounces boiling water

Juice from ½ lemon

Honey

Place the ginger and cinnamon in a mesh tea basket in a mug. Add the boiling water. Cover and steep for 10-15 minutes. Remove the tea basket and add the lemon juice and honey to taste. Alternatively, if slicing your ginger, you could skip the mesh strainer and let the ginger sink to the bottom of the mug; no need to strain.

Issues with Sperm and Testosterone

The strategies outlined in this book work together to enhance sperm quality, providing your best chance of pregnancy and a healthy baby. However, if sperm testing reveals significant issues with semen analysis or sperm DNA fragmentation, or it's taking longer to get pregnant than you are comfortable waiting, it's essential to investigate further.

The first step is to work with your doctor to rule out any serious conditions that may be hindering your fertility, such as infections, ejaculation issues, tumors, hormone imbalances, defects of the sperm transport tubes, or genetic conditions. It is also important to review with your doctor any medications you are taking, as some can impact sperm quality.

Once potential underlying conditions have been thoroughly investigated, you can discuss options and create a plan to support your fertility goals. Often a comprehensive evaluation may uncover a condition called varicocele.

Varicoceles

Varicoceles are enlarged veins in the scrotum, affecting roughly 15 percent of individuals with testicles. While many people may never notice them, for others, varicoceles can lead to fertility issues, reduced testosterone levels, or scrotal pain.

The exact ways varicoceles impact fertility aren't fully understood, but one significant factor is their effect on the temperature in the scrotum, where sperm and testosterone are produced. Normally, the testicles require a temperature about 2–4 degrees cooler than the body's average to function optimally. Varicoceles cause blood to pool in the scrotum, creating excess heat that can harm sperm and decrease testosterone production.

Diagnosing a varicocele typically involves a physical examination by a urologist. Larger varicoceles are often visible or can be felt, often described as feeling like a "bag of worms" in the scrotum. If a conclusive diagnosis cannot be made from a physical examination, a scrotal ultrasound may be ordered.

While varicoceles that aren't causing pain may not require treatment, repairing them surgically can often improve sperm quality, testosterone, and fertility. The procedure is relatively safe, so it's a good choice for people trying to have a baby naturally or through assisted reproductive procedures. People with extremely poor sperm concentrations and other egg or uterine factors might consider proceeding directly to IVF with ICSI in order to conceive.

After varicocele repair, sperm quality and testosterone levels often show improvement in about 3 months. During this time, it is helpful to support sperm production and healthy testosterone levels with the strategies discussed throughout this book, particularly:

Diet. Focus on antioxidant-rich fruits and veggies, reduce processed foods and alcohol, and maintain a healthy BMI (between 20 and 25).

Lifestyle. Keep the testicles cool by avoiding tight-fitting underwear and pants, hot tubs, saunas, long-distance biking, heated car seats, and sitting for long periods of time. Reduce your exposure to environmental chemicals (see Chapter 10).

Supplements. Consider incorporating supplements from Chapter 7, particularly vitamin D, omega-3 fatty acids, CoQ10, and a high-quality multivitamin.

Herbs. The following herbs from Chapter 8 can help improve sperm health: green tea, rooibos, turmeric, ashwagandha, maca, astragalus, and ginger. Don't forget to spice things up! Regularly incorporating herbs and spices in your meals is a great way to get more phytonutrients and antioxidants into your diet.

Combating Low Testosterone

Healthy testosterone levels are essential for sperm health, libido, erectile function, muscle mass, bone health, and feeling your best. While testosterone naturally declines with age, levels today are dropping faster than in previous generations, contributing to lower fertility rates.

The good news is that many factors affecting testosterone—such as nutrition, sleep, stress, and herbal support—are modifiable and respond well to targeted changes.

Nutrition. Ensure adequate intake of zinc, vitamin D, and magnesium while reducing alcohol consumption.

Movement. Resistance training and high-intensity interval training (HIIT) provide immediate and lasting benefits for testosterone levels.

Sleep. Poor sleep can lower testosterone by 10–15 percent after just 5 hours, and this reduction also disrupts sleep quality (see Chapter 9).

Stress. Chronic stress elevates cortisol, which suppresses testosterone (more in Chapter 9).

Herbs. Fenugreek (*Trigonella foenum-graecum*) in a dose of 500–600 mg daily is one of the best-researched herbs for boosting testosterone by reducing its conversion into estradiol and DHT. Other helpful herbs include ashwagandha, ginger, maca (Chapter 8), and reishi (Chapter 9).

Adopting these lifestyle and dietary strategies can significantly improve testosterone levels, fertility, and overall health.

CHAPTER 17

HERBAL SUPPORT

DURING FERTILITY TREATMENTS

······························

How to Safely Use Herbs Before and After Assisted Reproductive Technologies

Fertility treatments are a highly precise process where every element is carefully controlled. While some herbs provide supportive benefits, it's important to know what is safe to use and what should be avoided during this time.

When to Avoid Herbs and When to Return to Them

Assisted reproductive technologies (ARTs) are fertility treatments that include ovulation-stimulation medications (such as clomiphene [Clomid] and letrozole), intrauterine insemination (IUI), in vitro fertilization (IVF), and frozen embryo transfer (FET). The majority of herbs *should not be used during fertility treatments*, as they will have little or no effect in competition with fertility medications, and some could cause a negative interaction. If this is the road you choose, stop most of your herbal protocol and focus on the medical plan your doctor has outlined for you.

However, there are a handful of herbs that are completely safe and beneficial alongside ART fertility treatments. Included in this chapter is a breakdown of what herbs to safely reach for during the particular stages of fertility treatment.

Herbs During Medicated Fertility Cycles

When people describe their feelings at the beginning of their ART cycle, they say it resembles jumping onto a high-speed train, zooming through the countryside, over mountains, and under bridges. There's a whirlwind of activity, things are moving fast, and they don't always feel fully in control. The stakes are high, but they know the ultimate destination will be worth it . . . if they can get there.

During this time, you can safely support yourself with a little help from herbal allies.

Safe and gentle teas. Calming and nutritive herbs can provide much-needed support during the often stressful and uncertain ART process. Teas made from herbs like nettle, dandelion, rooibos, chamomile, lemon balm, peppermint, passionflower, and skullcap offer calming support and a boost of nutrition. They are safe during ART in standard amounts of 1–3 cups of tea made from one tea bag or up to approximately 1 tablespoon of herb per day. Green tea is also safe in standard amounts and offers a lower caffeine option than coffee.

Culinary herbs. Focus on the healthy food choices from Chapter 6 and culinary doses of fresh, garden herbs. These herbs, abundant in antioxidants and essential nutrients, contribute to overall health and wellness. Try adding a handful of greens like parsley, cilantro, and basil to any dish, and don't forget the spice rack for an added kick in taste and benefits!

Herbal Support During the 2-Week Wait

The "2-week wait" is the time after insemination or transfer when you are waiting until you can take a pregnancy test. Every minute of this time can be full of distraction, daydreaming, worry, and fear. After navigating the challenges of medications, injections, procedures, and testing, this period is a moment to catch your breath and surrender to the process. Remember, under normal circumstances, there's nothing you can do now to alter the outcome. It's time to focus on self-care: Prioritize sleep, nourish your body with wholesome foods, and nurture your nervous system.

Did you know that something as simple as mindfully preparing, holding, and sipping a cup of tea can have a calming effect on your mood? It's true! Studies have shown the benefits of this daily practice. During this waiting period, consider reaching for herbal teas like lemon balm and chamomile, known for their soothing properties. You can safely enjoy 1–3 cups of tea with these herbs a day.

Lemon balm (*Melissa officinalis*) is a mood-boosting hero of the herbal world. It can work quickly, quelling anxiety and lifting mood within an hour of ingesting. I particularly like lemon balm for times when you are feeling down, angry, or anxious—emotions so common during the 2-week wait.

Chamomile (*Matricaria chamomilla*) can help you wind down after a stressful day, particularly if you are prone to experiencing a "nervous stomach." Many people find chamomile's calming effects just enough to take the edge off. It is not too sedating to use during the day, but it is strong enough to help with insomnia in the evening. Avoid chamomile if you have a known allergy or react negatively to related plants, such as ragweed, chrysanthemums, marigolds, or daisies.

Daily De-Stress and Mood Lifter Tea

1 teaspoon dried peppermint
½ tablespoon dried chamomile flower
½ tablespoon dried lemon balm
8 ounces boiling water

Place the herbs in a mesh tea basket in a mug. Cover with the boiling water and steep for 5-15 minutes. Remove the tea basket and enjoy.

Herbal Support After an Unsuccessful ART Cycle

Everyone hopes that an IUI or IVF cycle works the first time, but that's not always the case. I know how it feels to have an unsuccessful IVF cycle—I've been through three myself. I remember how uncomfortable and bloated my body felt, and how emotional the whole process was for me. Looking back, I realize the importance of having a support plan in place to nurture both my body and my mind during such challenging times.

A supportive plan following an unsuccessful ART cycle typically includes gentle support for the liver and nervous system.

Gentle Liver Support

Think of the liver as the body's chemical processing plant and housekeeper. It metabolizes our hormones, medications, and other toxins and packages them up into compounds that can be released through urine or stool. Ideally, when everything's running smoothly, your liver efficiently processes these substances, allowing you to eliminate them every time you pee and have a bowel movement.

During ART cycles, medication and elevated hormone levels have the liver working overtime. While the liver is perfectly capable of handling this extra demand, you can help by providing the raw materials the liver relies on to do its job more efficiently. It's also important to address constipation, which can be a common side effect of IVF. If you're not pooping every day, toxins and old hormones may linger in your system, potentially leading to their reabsorption and circulation throughout the body.

First things first: Deal with constipation if that is an issue for you!

It's essential to keep things moving, with the goal of at least one bowel movement every day. After ART treatments, the abdominal area can be bloated and feel tender. Constipation will only contribute to feeling uncomfortable and get in the way of your liver's natural detoxification process. Remember, it's important to make sure you are eliminating the toxins that the liver is breaking down, so if you are even a little bit constipated, be proactive and take steps to stay regular.

Strategies to manage constipation:

- Drink plenty of water.

- Start your day with warm lemon water: 8 ounces of warm water and the juice of ½ lemon.

- Drink 1–2 cups of Lemon Ginger Tea (see page 102) throughout the day.

- Short-term use of herbal tea with gentle laxative action. If the first three suggestions aren't enough to get things moving again after 1–2 days, try a gentle herbal laxative tea.

Next, support the liver's natural detoxification process.

Detoxification is a very nutrient-demanding process. The liver relies heavily on a steady supply of B vitamins, antioxidants, and protein to do its job effectively, so it's essential to ensure you're getting all the goodies your liver craves. If you're already enjoying a well-rounded diet and sticking to your prenatal multivitamin routine, you're likely on the right track. Now's not the time for drastic cleanses or dietary restrictions. Instead, consider incorporating liver-supportive herbs to give your liver a little extra love.

Strategies to support the liver:

- Continue eating lots of fruits, veggies, and adequate protein (refer to Chapter 6 for more details).

- Continue taking your prenatal multivitamins.

- Limit or avoid alcohol, as alcohol can be an additional stressor for your liver.

Herbal teas to bump up antioxidants and vitamins. Every herb listed in Chapter 8 would fit the bill here! One of my favorite herbal recipes is the Overnight Nettle and Oat Straw Infusion (see page 92)—a nutritive blend full of antioxidants, vitamins, and minerals. Make a batch in the evening, let it steep overnight, and drink over the next 1–2 days.

Herbal teas that gently increase liver detoxification. Many herbs can be helpful to support liver detoxification and are gentle and safe even if you are planning on going right into another ART cycle. These herbs can be taken from the time you have a negative pregnancy test until you start your next round of medications: dandelion root, schisandra berry (Chapter 9), turmeric (Chapter 8), and ginger (Chapter 8). One of my favorite herbal drinks for a little extra liver support is golden milk (see the recipe on page 94). The star ingredient in golden milk is turmeric, which is high in antioxidants and helps with liver detoxification.

Nervous System Support

Undergoing ART treatments is undeniably taxing, both physically and emotionally. Scheduling some downtime following your ART cycle provides the
necessary breathing room for whatever lies ahead on your journey. Rather
than powering through, prioritize giving yourself the opportunity to heal and
recharge, ensuring you're in a better place, both mentally and physically, for
whatever comes next.

Herbal teas offer a remarkable way to navigate the emotional challenges of
heartbreak, grief, fear, uncertainty, and anxiety. While all the herbs discussed in
the Chapter 9 section Stress Is Real are beneficial, here are a few client favorites.

Lemon Balm Tea. Brew a comforting cup by adding 1 heaping teaspoon of
dried lemon balm to boiling water. Let it steep for 10–15 minutes, then savor.
For added convenience, organic tea bags are readily available.

Daily De-Stress and Mood Lifter Tea. This uplifting yet calming tea, fea-
tured on page 178, provides a soothing pick-me-up during stressful times.

Schisandra Berry Lemon Balm Tea. Combine the mood-enhancing properties of lemon balm with the de-stressing effects of schisandra berry in this
delightful tea described below. Not only does it lift spirits and promote relaxation, but schisandra also supports liver detoxification.

Schisandra Berry Lemon Balm Tea

1 tablespoon dried lemon balm
1 teaspoon dried schisandra berries
8 ounces boiling water
Honey (optional)

Combine the lemon balm and schisandra in a mesh tea basket in a mug.
Add the boiling water. Cover and steep for 10-15 minutes. Remove the tea
basket, add honey to taste, if desired, and enjoy.

While herbal remedies are invaluable, healing and recovery extend beyond
botanical support alone. Tune in to your body's signals—what does it crave right
now? Whether it's more rest, meaningful connections with loved ones, or quiet
moments for introspection and processing, honor those needs without judgment. The aim is to transition from a state of heightened stress to one of calm
and stability.

Here are a few ideas.

- Prioritize sleep.
- Practice breathing exercises.
- Engage in meditation.
- Explore journaling.
- Spend time in nature.
- Enjoy adult coloring.
- Try tapping techniques.

Remember, you don't need to incorporate every suggestion into your routine. Simply select one that resonates with you as a starting point for nurturing your body.

AFTERWORD

The Herbal Fertility Holistic Approach

While quick fixes and miracle remedies may be tempting, true fertility support is deeper than single solutions. My hope for you, after reading this book, is that you now understand there is no magic bullet to help you reach your end goal of getting pregnant.

The intention of *The Herbal Fertility Handbook* is to provide suggestions, tips, and answers about herbs and lifestyle changes that will enhance egg quality, regulate menstrual cycles, and turn sperm into super swimmers.

Within these pages is a wealth of tools to dramatically support and shift your fertility journey. Woven together, the solutions are surprisingly simple, drawing from centuries of wisdom and validated by modern science. In today's fast-paced world, we often lose touch with the natural rhythms that support our fertility. At the heart of the holistic fertility approach are the herbs. More than just their individual chemical constituents, whole-plant herbs offer opportunities for vibrant health and fertility. Incorporating herbs into daily life, whether as seasonings or in tinctures, teas, and capsules, provides essential and often missing elements from plants that our bodies need.

Now you know how important it is to slow down, live a lifestyle where you prioritize restful sleep and energizing movement, nourish your body with whole foods, embrace the healing power of herbs, and remove harmful chemicals and toxins from our bodies, all to create a space to thrive and welcome a tiny new human.

Let's reflect on Jack and Emily's fertility journeys.

When Jack and his partner initially sought my assistance, they were struggling with the diagnosis of unexplained infertility. When we dug into Jack's semen analysis and viewed it through the lens of what is optimal versus what is normal, it became clear that Jack's sperm parameters could use some support. We put a plan in place that focused on sperm health, taking into consideration Jack's stress levels and sleep struggles. A few weeks after starting the protocol, Jack was falling asleep easier and sleeping through most nights. His stress levels at work felt lower, and he was feeling less anxious overall. Over the next 3 months, he felt more energized. The plan was to repeat the semen analysis at the 6-month mark, but Jack and his partner were pregnant by month 4! They went on to have a happy, healthy baby and continued to incorporate many of the strategies they'd learned to support their overall health and wellness.

Emily was not content to simply take a prenatal vitamin and try for 1 year. At 34 years old, she was committed to maximizing her chances of conceiving and having a healthy baby. Her strategy focused on incorporating plenty of antioxidants, targeted supplements, and gentle herbs into her routine. Over time, Emily experienced a significant improvement in her painful periods, which she had previously accepted as normal. Meditation and regular physical activity became integral parts of her daily life, making the stress of her fertility journey more manageable. Just 5 months after implementing her protocol, Emily and her partner received the joyful news of pregnancy. Today their baby is a happy and healthy toddler. The combination of nutritional strategies, herbal teas, and stress management techniques provided a sturdy foundation that Emily continued to help her navigate the postpartum and new parent landscape.

This book is your invitation and guide to embrace a holistic approach to fertility—one that harnesses the power of nature while integrating the advancements of science, diagnostic testing, and reproductive technologies. It's a journey of discovery, empowerment, and profound connection—to yourself, to the world around you, and to the possibility of new life.

GRATITUDE AND ACKNOWLEDGMENTS

Herbal medicine is based on the traditions and knowledge of Indigenous peoples worldwide. It has been passed down through generations and forms the foundation of modern herbalism. It is with profound respect and gratitude that I honor this wisdom and the healing power of the plants themselves.

I am incredibly grateful to the many herbalists who have shared their knowledge with me over the years—some I've had the privilege to learn from personally and some whose wisdom has reached me through books, lectures, and podcasts.

To my first and most influential teacher, Maria Noël Groves, thank you for sharing both your love of plants and your vast clinical experience. Your ability to blend traditional herbal wisdom with the latest scientific research has profoundly shaped my practice. I am also grateful for your encouragement and support throughout the writing of this book.

To Camille Freeman, thank you for creating a supportive community where herbalists can continue to learn and grow together. Your guidance and encouragement have been invaluable in writing this book.

My heartfelt thanks to the herbalists who have made a lasting impact on our field, whose work has informed my practice and continues to inspire me: Rosemary Gladstar; David Winston; Aviva Romm, MD; Rosalee de la Forêt; Thomas Easley; Jill Stansbury, ND; and Kat Maier, to name a few.

Thank you to the clients who have shared their journeys with me, allowing me to play a role in their stories, their fertility, and their families.

I am forever grateful to my husband, whose support and encouragement has never wavered.

And most importantly, to my twin, teenage daughters—it was my own personal journey to your conception that has shaped our family, my career, and has ultimately led to the publication of this book. Thank you for letting me discuss sperm, eggs, menstrual cycles, and all things fertility without too much embarrassment!

Resources

Here are some trusted companies, organizations, and guides that I hope will support you in your fertility journey.

LOOSE-LEAF HERBS AND POWDERS

Banyan Botanicals
https://banyanbotanicals.com

Foster Farm Botanicals
https://fosterfarmbotanicals.com
/collections/botanicals

Mountain Rose Herbs
https://mountainroseherbs.com

Oshala Farm
https://oshalafarm.com

Zack Woods Herb Farm
https://zackwoodsherbs.com

TEA BAGS

Mountain Rose Herbs
https://mountainroseherbs.com

Numi
https://numitea.com

Organic India
https://organicindiausa.com

Traditional Medicinals
https://traditionalmedicinals.com

HERBAL TINCTURES

Avena Botanicals
https://avenabotanicals.com

Gaia Herbs
https://gaiaherbs.com

Herbalist & Alchemist
https://herbalist-alchemist.com

Herb Pharm
https://herb-pharm.com

Mountain Rose Herbs
https://mountainroseherbs.com

Wise Woman Herbals
https://wisewomanherbals.com

HERBAL CAPSULES

Gaia Herbs
https://gaiaherbs.com

Herbalist & Alchemist
https://herbalist-alchemist.com

Oregon's Wild Harvest
https://oregonswildharvest.com

SUPPORT GROUPS

AllPaths Family Building
https://allpathsfb.org

RESOLVE: The National Fertility Association
https://resolve.org

EDUCATION AND GUIDES

Environmental Working Group
https://ewg.org

EWG Tap Water Database
https://ewg.org/tapwater

EWG's Skin Deep Cosmetics Database
https://ewg.org/skindeep

EWG's Cleaning Products Guide
https://ewg.org/cleaners

References

CHAPTER 1

1. Lepkowski, J. M., Mosher, W. D., Davis, K. E., Groves, R. M., & Van Hoewyk, J. (2010). The 2006–2010 National Survey of Family Growth: Sample design and analysis of a continuous survey. *Vital and Health Statistics, 2*(150). https://www.cdc.gov /nchs/data/series/sr_02/sr02_150.pdf

CHAPTER 2

1. Fragouli, E., Alfarawati, S., Goodall, N. N., Sánchez-García, J. F., Colls, P., & Wells, D. (2011). The cytogenetics of polar bodies: Insights into female meiosis and the diagnosis of aneuploidy. *MHR: Basic Science of Reproductive Medicine, 17*(5), 286–295. https://doi.org/10.1093/molehr /gar024

2. Horan, C. J., & Williams, S. A. (2017). Oocyte stem cells: Fact or fantasy? *Reproduction (Cambridge, England), 154*(1), R23–R35. https://doi.org/10.1530/REP-17-0008

3. Bull, J. R., Rowland, S. P., Scherwitzl, E. B., Scherwitzl, R., Danielsson, K. G., & Harper, J. (2019). Real-world menstrual cycle characteristics of more than 600,000 menstrual cycles. *NPJ Digital Medicine, 2*(1), 83. https://doi: 10.1038 /s41746-019-0152-7

CHAPTER 3

1. Yatsenko, A. N., & Turek, P. J. (2018). Reproductive genetics and the aging male. *Journal of Assisted Reproduction and Genetics, 35*, 933–941. https://doi.org/10.1007/s10815-018-1148-y

CHAPTER 4

1. Johnson, S., Weddell, S., Godbert, S., Freundl, G., Roos, J., & Gnoth, C. (2015). Development of the first urinary reproductive hormone ranges referenced to independently determined ovulation day. *Clinical Chemistry and Laboratory Medicine (CCLM), 53*(7), 1099–1108. https://doi.org/10.1515 /cclm-2014-1087

2. Wilcox, A. J., Weinberg, C. R., & Baird, D. D. (1995). Timing of sexual intercourse in relation to ovulation—effects on the probability of conception, survival of the pregnancy, and sex of the baby. *New England Journal of Medicine, 333*(23), 1517–1521.

3. Levitas, E., Lunenfeld, E., Weiss, N., Friger, M., Har-Vardi, I., Koifman, A., & Potashnik, G. (2005). Relationship between the duration of sexual abstinence and semen quality: Analysis of 9,489 semen samples. *Fertility and Sterility, 83*(6), 1680–1686. https://doi.org/10.1016/j.fertnstert.2004.12.045

4. Check, J. H., Epstein, R., & Long, R. (1991). Effect of time interval between ejaculations on semen parameters. *Archives of Andrology, 27*(2), 93–95. https://doi.org/10.3109/01485019108987658

CHAPTER 5

1. World Health Organization. (2010). *WHO Laboratory Manual for the Examination and Processing of Human Semen* (5th ed.). Retrieved from https://www.who.int/docs/default-source /reproductive-health/srhr-documents/infertility /examination-and-processing-of-human-semen -5ed-eng.pdf

2. Cooper, T. G., Noonan, E., von Eckardstein, S., Auger, J., Gordon Baker, H. W., Behre, H. M., . . . Vogelsong, K. M. (2010). World Health Organization reference values for human semen characteristics. *Human Reproduction Update, 16*(3), 231–245. https://doi.org/10.1093/humupd/dmp048

3. Wang, C., & Swerdloff, R. S. (2014). Limitations of semen analysis as a test of male fertility and anticipated needs from newer tests. *Fertility and Sterility, 102*(6), 1502–1507. https://doi.org/10.1016 /j.fertnstert.2014.10.021

4. Butcher, M. J., Janoo, J., Broce, M., Seybold, D. J., Gantt, P., & Randall, G. (2016). Use of sperm parameters to predict clinical pregnancy with intrauterine insemination. *Journal of Reproductive Medicine, 61*(5–6), 263–269.

5. Levine, H., Jørgensen, N., Martino-Andrade, A., Mendiola, J., Weksler-Derri, D., Mindlis, I., . . . Swan, S. H. (2017). Temporal trends in sperm count: A systematic review and meta-regression analysis. *Human Reproduction Update, 23*(6), 646–659. https://doi.org/10.1093/humupd/dmx022

6. Tiegs, A. W., Landis, J., Garrido, N., Scott, R. T. Jr., & Hotaling, J. M. (2019). Total motile sperm count trend over time: Evaluation of semen analyses from 119,972 men from subfertile couples. *Urology, 132*, 109–116. https://doi.org/10.1016 /j.urology.2019.06.038

7. Chang, S., Nazem, T. G., Gounko, D., Lee, J., Bar-Chama, N., Shamonki, J. M., . . . Copperman, A. B. (2018). Eleven year longitudinal study of US sperm donors demonstrates declining sperm count and motility. *Fertility and Sterility*, *110*(4), e54–e55. https://doi.org/10.1016/j.fertnstert.2018.07.170

8. Carlsen, E., Giwercman, A., Keiding, N., & Skakkebaek, N. E. (1992). Evidence for decreasing quality of semen during past 50 years. *British Medical Journal*, *305*(6854), 609–613. https://doi.org/10.1136/bmj.305.6854.609

9. Bonde, J. P., Ernst, E., Jensen, T. K., Hjollund, N. H., Kolstad, H., Scheike, T., . . . Olsen, J. (1998). Relation between semen quality and fertility: A population-based study of 430 first-pregnancy planners. *Lancet*, *352*(9135), 1172–1177. https://doi.org/10.1016/S0140-6736(97)10514-1

10. Skakkebaek, N. E., Lindahl-Jacobsen, R., Levine, H., Andersson, A. M., Jørgensen, N., Main, K. M., . . . Juul, A. (2022). Environmental factors in declining human fertility. *Nature Reviews Endocrinology*, *18*(3), 139–157. https://doi.org/10.1038/s41574-021-00598-8

11. Kortenkamp, A., Scholze, M., Ermler, S., Priskorn, L., Jørgensen, N., Andersson, A. M., & Frederiksen, H. (2022). Combined exposures to bisphenols, polychlorinated dioxins, paracetamol, and phthalates as drivers of deteriorating semen quality. *Environment International*, *165*, 107322. https://doi.org/10.1016/j.envint.2022.107322

12. Aitken, R. J. (2017). Reactive oxygen species as mediators of sperm capacitation and pathological damage. *Molecular Reproduction and Development*, *84*(10), 1039–1052. https://doi.org/10.1002/mrd.22871

13. Meseguer, M., Santiso, R., Garrido, N., García-Herrero, S., Remohí, J., & Fernandez, J. L. (2011). Effect of sperm DNA fragmentation on pregnancy outcome depends on oocyte quality. *Fertility and Sterility*, *95*(1), 124–128. https://doi.org/10.1016/j.fertnstert.2010.05.055

CHAPTER 6

1. Bird, J. K., Murphy, R. A., Ciappio, E. D., & McBurney, M. I. (2017). Risk of deficiency in multiple concurrent micronutrients in children and adults in the United States. *Nutrients*, *9*(7), 655. https://doi.org/10.3390/nu9070655

2. Zhang, Y., Zhang, J., Zhao, J., Hong, X., Zhang, H., Dai, Q., . . . Ma, X. (2020). Couples' prepregnancy body mass index and time to pregnancy among those attempting to conceive their first pregnancy. *Fertility and Sterility*, *114*(5), 1067–1075. https://doi.org/10.1016/j.fertnstert.2020.05.041

3. Osadchiy, V., Belarmino, A., Kianian, R., Sigalos, J. T., Ancira, J. S., Kanie, T., . . . Eleswarapu, S. V. (2024). Semen microbiota are dramatically altered in men with abnormal sperm parameters. *Scientific Reports*, *14*(1), 1068.

4. Al-Nasiry, S., Ambrosino, E., Schlaepfer, M., Morré, S. A., Wieten, L., Voncken, J. W., . . . Kramer, B. W. (2020). The interplay between reproductive tract microbiota and immunological system in human reproduction. *Frontiers in Immunology*, *11*, 378. https://doi.org/10.3389/fimmu.2020.00378

5. Liu, J., Liu, Y., & Li, X. (2023). Effects of intestinal flora on polycystic ovary syndrome. *Frontiers in Endocrinology*, *14*, 1151723. https://doi.org/10.3389/fendo.2023.1151723

6. Bear, T., Dalziel, J., Coad, J., Roy, N., Butts, C., & Gopal, P. (2021). The microbiome-gut-brain axis and resilience to developing anxiety or depression under stress. *Microorganisms*, *9*(4), 723. https://doi.org/10.3390/microorganisms9040723

7. Li, Y., Hao, Y., Fan, F., & Zhang, B. (2018). The role of microbiome in insomnia, circadian disturbance and depression. *Frontiers in Psychiatry, 9*. https://doi.org/10.3389/fpsyt.2018.00669

8. Hua, X., Cao, Y., Morgan, D. M., Miller, K., Chin, S. M., Bellavance, D., & Khalili, H. (2022). Longitudinal analysis of the impact of oral contraceptive use on the gut microbiome. *Journal of Medical Microbiology*, *71*(4). https://doi.org/10.1099/jmm.0.001512

9. Kazi, Y. F., Saleem, S., & Kazi, N. (2012). Investigation of vaginal microbiota in sexually active women using hormonal contraceptives in Pakistan. *BMC Urology*, *12*(1), 1–5. https://doi.org/10.1186/1471-2490-12-22

10. Suez, J., Cohen, Y., Valdés-Mas, R., Mor, U., Dori-Bachash, M., Federici, S., . . . Elinav, E. (2022). Personalized microbiome-driven effects of non-nutritive sweeteners on human glucose tolerance. *Cell*, *185*(18), 3307–3328. https://doi.org/10.1016/j.cell.2022.07.016

11. Tun, H. M., Konya, T., Takaro, T. K., Brook, J. R., Chari, R., Field, C. J., . . . & Kozyrskyj, A. L. (2017). Exposure to household furry pets influences the gut microbiota of infants at 3–4 months following various birth scenarios. *Microbiome, 5*, 1–14. https://doi.org/10.1186/s40168-017-0254-x

12. Çekici, H., & Akdevelioğlu, Y. (2019). The association between trans fatty acids, infertility and fetal life: A review. *Human Fertility* (Cambridge, England), *22*(3), 154–163. https://doi.org/10.1080/14647273.2018.1432078

13. Chavarro, J. E., Rich-Edwards, J. W., Rosner, B. A., & Willett, W. C. (2007). Dietary fatty acid intakes and the risk of ovulatory infertility. *American Journal of Clinical Nutrition, 85*(1), 231–237. https://doi.org/10.1093/ajcn/85.1.231

14. Hatch, E. E., Wise, L. A., Mikkelsen, E. M., Christensen, T., Riis, A. H., Sørensen, H. T., & Rothman, K. J. (2012). Caffeinated beverage and soda consumption and time to pregnancy. *Epidemiology (Cambridge, Mass.), 23*(3), 393. https://doi.org/10.1097/EDE.0b013e31824cbaac

15. Hatch, E. E., Wesselink, A. K., Hahn, K. A., Michiel, J. J., Mikkelsen, E. M., Sorensen, H. T., . . . Wise, L. A. (2018). Intake of sugar-sweetened beverages and fecundability in a North American preconception cohort. *Epidemiology (Cambridge, Mass.), 29*(3), 369. https://doi.org/10.1097/EDE.0000000000000812

16. Setti, A. S., Braga, D. P. D. A. F., Halpern, G., Rita de Cássia, S. F., Iaconelli, A. Jr., & Borges, E., Jr. (2018). Is there an association between artificial sweetener consumption and assisted reproduction outcomes? *Reproductive Biomedicine Online, 36*(2), 145–153. https://doi.org/10.1016/j.rbmo.2017.11.004

17. Lyngsø, J., Kesmodel, U. S., Bay, B., Ingerslev, H. J., Andersen, A. M. N., & Ramlau-Hansen, C. H. (2019). Impact of female daily coffee consumption on successful fertility treatment: A Danish cohort study. *Fertility and Sterility, 112*(1), 120–129. https://doi.org/10.1016/j.fertnstert.2019.03.014

CHAPTER 7

1. Doguc, D. K., Deniz, F., İlhan, İ., Ergonul, E., & Gultekin, F. (2021). Prenatal exposure to artificial food colorings alters NMDA receptor subunit concentrations in rat hippocampus. *Nutritional Neuroscience, 24*(10), 784–794. https://doi.org/10.1080/1028415X.2019.1681065

2. Miller, M. D., Steinmaus, C., Golub, M. S., Castorina, R., Thilakartne, R., Bradman, A., & Marty, M. A. (2022). Potential impacts of synthetic food dyes on activity and attention in children: A review of the human and animal evidence. *Environmental Health, 21*(1), 45. https://doi.org/10.1186/s12940-022-00849-9

3. Tucker, J., Fischer, T., Upjohn, L., Mazzera, D., & Kumar, M. (2018). Unapproved pharmaceutical ingredients included in dietary supplements associated with US Food and Drug Administration warnings. *JAMA Network Open, 1*(6), e183337. https://doi.org/10.1001/jamanetworkopen.2018.3337

4. Crider, K. S., Zhu, J. H., Hao, L., Yang, Q. H., Yang, T. P., Gindler, J., . . . Berry, R. J. (2011). MTHFR 677C->T genotype is associated with folate and homocysteine concentrations in a large, population-based, double-blind trial of folic acid supplementation. *American Journal of Clinical Nutrition, 93*(6), 1365–1372. https://doi.org/10.3945/ajcn.110.004671

5. Palacios, A. M., Feiner, R. A., & Cabrera, R. M. (2023). Characterization of folic acid, 5-methyltetrahydrofolate and synthetic folinic acid in the high-affinity folate transporters: Impact on pregnancy and development. *Reproductive and Developmental Medicine, 7*(02), 102–107.

6. Chu, J., Gallos, I., Tobias, A., Tan, B., Eapen, A., & Coomarasamy, A. (2018). Vitamin D and assisted reproductive treatment outcome: A systematic review and meta-analysis. *Human Reproduction, 33*(1), 65–80. https://doi.org/10.1093/humrep/dex326

7. Rudick, B. J., Ingles, S. A., Chung, K., Stanczyk, F. Z., Paulson, R. J., & Bendikson, K. A. (2014). Influence of vitamin D levels on in vitro fertilization outcomes in donor-recipient cycles. *Fertility and Sterility, 101*(2), 447–452. https://doi.org/10.1016/j.fertnstert.2013.10.008

8. Mumford, S. L., Garbose, R. A., Kim, K., Kissell, K., Kuhr, D. L., Omosigho, U. R., . . . Schisterman, E. F. (2018). Association of preconception serum 25-hydroxyvitamin D concentrations with livebirth and pregnancy loss: A prospective cohort study. *Lancet. Diabetes & Endocrinology, 6*(9), 725–732. https://doi.org/10.1016/S2213-8587(18)30153-0

9. Stanhiser, J., Jukic, A. M. Z., McConnaughey, D. R., & Steiner, A. Z. (2022). Omega-3 fatty acid supplementation and fecundability. *Human Reproduction (Oxford, England), 37*(5), 1037–1046. https://doi.org/10.1093/humrep/deac027

10. Chiu, Y. H., Karmon, A. E., Gaskins, A. J., Arvizu, M., Williams, P. L., Souter, I., . . . EARTH Study Team. (2018). Serum omega-3 fatty acids and treatment outcomes among women undergoing assisted reproduction. *Human Reproduction, 33*(1), 156–165. https://doi.org/10.1093/humrep/dex335

11. Yang, L., Wang, H., Song, S., Xu, H., Chen, Y., Tian, S., . . . Zhang, Q. (2022). Systematic understanding of anti-aging effect of coenzyme Q10 on oocyte through a network pharmacology approach. *Frontiers in Endocrinology, 13*, 813772. https://doi.org/10.3389/fendo.2022.813772

12. Safarinejad, M. R. (2011). Effect of omega-3 polyunsaturated fatty acid supplementation on semen profile and enzymatic anti-oxidant capacity of seminal plasma in infertile men with idiopathic oligoasthenoteratospermia: A double-blind, placebo-controlled, randomised study. *Andrologia, 43*(1), 38–47. https://doi .org/10.1111/j.1439-0272.2009.01013.x

13. Martínez-Soto, J. C., Domingo, J. C., Cordobilla, B., Nicolás, M., Fernández, L., Albero, P., . . .Landeras, J. (2016). Dietary supplementation with docosahexaenoic acid (DHA) improves sem-inal antioxidant status and decreases sperm DNA fragmentation. *Systems Biology in Reproductive Medicine, 62*(6), 387–395. https://doi.org/10.1080 /19396368.2016.1246623

14. Robbins, W. A., Xun, L., FitzGerald, L. Z., Esguerra, S., Henning, S. M., & Carpenter, C. L. (2012). Walnuts improve semen quality in men consuming a Western-style diet: Randomized control dietary intervention trial. *Biology of Reproduction, 87*(4), 101. https://doi.org /10.1095/biolreprod.112.101634

15. Balercia, G., Mancini, A., Paggi, F., Tiano, L., Pontecorvi, A., Boscaro, M., . . . Littarru, G. P. (2009). Coenzyme Q10 and male infertility. *Journal of Endocrinological Investigation, 32*(7), 626–632. https://doi.org/10.1007/BF03346521

16. Tania, C., Tobing, E. R. P. L., Tansol, C., Prasetiyo, P. D., Wallad, C. K., & Hariyanto, T. I. (2023). Vitamin D supplementation for improving sperm parameters in infertile men: A systematic review and meta-analysis of randomized clinical trials. *Arab Journal of Urology*, 1–9.

17. Güngör, K., Güngör, N. D., Başar, M. M., Cengiz, F., Erşahin, S. S., & Çil, K. (2022). Relationship between serum vitamin D levels semen parameters and sperm DNA damage in men with unexplained infertility. *European Review for Medical and Pharmacological Sciences, 26*(2), 499–505. https://doi.org/10.26355/eurrev_ 202201_27875

18. Lerchbaum, E., Pilz, S., Trummer, C., Rabe, T., Schenk, M., Heijboer, A. C., & Obermayer-Pietsch, B. (2014). Serum vitamin D levels and hypogonad-ism in men. *Andrology, 2*(5), 748–754. https://doi.org/10.1111/j.2047-2927.2014.00247.x

CHAPTER 8

1. Zhang, Y., Lin, H., Liu, C., Huang, J., & Liu, Z. (2020). A review for physiological activities of EGCG and the role in improving fertility in humans/ mammals. *Biomedicine & Pharmacotherapy, 127*, 110186. https://doi.org/10.1016/j.biopha.2020 .110186

2. Fukushima, Y., Ohie, T., Yonekawa, Y., Yonemoto, K., Aizawa, H., Mori, Y., . . . Kondo, K. (2009). Coffee and green tea are a large source of anti-oxidant polyphenols in the Japanese population. *Journal of Agricultural and Food Chemistry, 57*(4), 1253–1259. https://doi.org/10.1021/jf802418j

3. Rahman, S. U., Huang, Y., Zhu, L., Feng, S., Khan, I. M., Wu, J., . . . Wang, X. (2018). Therapeutic role of green tea polyphenols in improving fertility: A review. *Nutrients, 10*(7), 834. https://doi.org/10.3390/nu10070834

4. Roychoudhury, S., Agarwal, A., Virk, G., & Cho, C. L. (2017). Potential role of green tea catechins in the management of oxidative stress-associated infertility. *Reproductive Biomedicine Online, 34*(5), 487–498. https://doi.org/10.1016 /j.rbmo.2017.02.006

5. De Amicis, F., Santoro, M., Guido, C., Russo, A., & Aquila, S. (2012). Epigallocatechin gallate affects survival and metabolism of human sperm. *Molecular Nutrition & Food Research, 56*(11), 1655–1664. https://doi.org/10.1002 /mnfr.201200190

6. See note 4.

7. Oketch-Rabah, H. A., Roe, A. L., Rider, C. V., Bonkovsky, H. L., Giancaspro, G. I., Navarro, V., . . . & Ko, R. (2020). United States Pharmacopeia (USP) comprehensive review of the hepatotoxicity of green tea extracts. *Toxicology Reports, 7*, 386–402. https://doi.org/10.1016/j.toxrep.2020.02.008

8. Yan, K., Qie, Z., Vásquez, E., Guo, F., Zhang, L., Lin, Z., & Qin, H. (2022). Tea consumption during the periconceptional period does not significantly increase the prevalence of neural tube defects: A systematic review and dose-response meta-analysis. *Nutrition Research (New York, NY), 102*, 13–22. https://doi.org/10.1016 /j.nutres.2022.02.009

9. Jia, X., Ren, M., Zhang, Y., Ye, R., Zhang, L., & Li, Z. (2021). Association between tea drinking and plasma folate concentration among women aged 18–30 years in China. *Public Health Nutrition, 24*(15), 4929–4936.

10. Awoniyi, D. O., Aboua, Y. G., Marnewick, J., & Brooks, N. (2012). The effects of rooibos (*Aspalathus linearis*), green tea (*Camellia sinensis*) and commercial rooibos and green tea supplements on epididymal sperm in oxidative stress-induced rats. *Phytotherapy Research: PTR, 26*(8), 1231–1239. https://doi.org/10.1002/ptr.3717

11. Sirotkin A. V. (2022). Rooibos (*Aspalathus linearis*) influence on health and ovarian functions. *Journal of Animal Physiology and Animal Nutrition, 106*(5), 995–999. https://doi.org/10.1111/jpn.13624

12. Gammoudi, B. K. (2019). Evaluating the neuroprotective effects of fermented rooibos herbal tea in Wistar rats exposed to bisphenol-a during gestation and lactation. https://core.ac.uk/reader/199461330

13. Alizadeh, F., Javadi, M., Karami, A. A., Gholaminejad, F., Kavianpour, M., & Haghighian, H. K. (2018). Curcumin nanomicelle improves semen parameters, oxidative stress, inflammatory biomarkers, and reproductive hormones in infertile men: A randomized clinical trial. *Phytotherapy Research, 32*(3), 514–521. https://doi.org/10.1002/ptr.5998

14. Zhang, L., Diao, R. Y., Duan, Y. G., Yi, T. H., & Cai, Z. M. (2017). In vitro antioxidant effect of curcumin on human sperm quality in leucocytospermia. *Andrologia, 49*(10), e12760. https://doi.org/10.1111/and.12760

15. Zhou, Q., Wu, X., Liu, Y., Wang, X., Ling, X., Ge, H., & Zhang, J. (2020). Curcumin improves asthenozoospermia by inhibiting reactive oxygen species reproduction through nuclear factor erythroid 2-related factor 2 activation. *Andrologia, 52*(2), e13491. https://doi.org/10.1111/and.13491

16. Campbell, M. S., Carlini, N. A., & Fleenor, B. S. (2021). Influence of curcumin on performance and post-exercise recovery. *Critical Reviews in Food Science and Nutrition, 61*(7), 1152–1162. https://doi.org/10.1080/10408398.2020.1754754

17. Naz, R. K., & Lough, M. L. (2014). Curcumin as a potential non-steroidal contraceptive with spermicidal and microbicidal properties. *European Journal of Obstetrics & Gynecology and Reproductive Biology, 176*, 142–148.

18. Głombik, K., Basta-Kaim, A., Sikora-Polaczek, M., Kubera, M., Starowicz, G., & Styrna, J. (2014). Curcumin influences semen quality parameters and reverses the di(2-ethylhexyl)phthalate (DEHP)-induced testicular damage in mice. *Pharmacological Reports: PR, 66*(5), 782–787. https://doi.org/10.1016/j.pharep.2014.04.010

19. Mishra, R. K., & Singh, S. K. (2009). Reversible antifertility effect of aqueous rhizome extract of *Curcuma longa* L. in male laboratory mice. *Contraception, 79*(6), 479–487. https://doi.org/10.1016/j.contraception.2009.01.001

20. Ashok, P., & Meenakshi, B. (2004). Contraceptive effect of *Curcuma longa* (L.) in male albino rats. *Asian Journal of Andrology, 6*(1), 71–74.

21. Mahdi, A. A., Shukla, K. K., Ahmad, M. K., Rajender, S., Shankhwar, S. N., Singh, V., & Dalela, D. (2011). *Withania somnifera* improves semen quality in stress-related male fertility. *Evidence-Based Complementary and Alternative Medicine, 2011*, Article ID 576962. https://doi.org/10.1093/ecam/nep138

22. Ambiye, V. R., Langade, D., Dongre, S., Aptikar, P., Kulkarni, M., & Dongre, A. (2013). Clinical evaluation of the spermatogenic activity of the root extract of ashwagandha (*Withania somnifera*) in oligospermic males: A pilot study. *Evidence-Based Complementary and Alternative Medicine, 2013*, Article ID 571420. https://doi.org/10.1155/2013/571420

23. Ahmad, M. K., Mahdi, A. A., Shukla, K. K., Islam, N., Rajender, S., Madhukar, D., . . . Ahmad, S. (2010). *Withania somnifera* improves semen quality by regulating reproductive hormone levels and oxidative stress in seminal plasma of infertile males. *Fertility and Sterility, 94*(3), 989–996. https://doi.org/10.1016/j.fertnstert.2009.04.046

24. Ambiye, V. R., Langade, D., Dongre, S., Aptikar, P., Kulkarni, M., & Dongre, A. (2013). Clinical evaluation of the spermatogenic activity of the root extract of ashwagandha (*Withania somnifera*) in oligospermic males: A pilot study. *Evidence-Based Complementary and Alternative Medicine, 2013*, Article ID 571420. https://doi.org/10.1155/2013/571420

25. Chauhan, S., Srivastava, M. K., & Pathak, A. K. (2022). Effect of standardized root extract of ashwagandha (*Withania somnifera*) on well-being and sexual performance in adult males: A randomized controlled trial. *Health Science Reports, 5*(4), e741. https://doi.org/10.1002/hsr2.741

26. Gonzales, G. F., Córdova, A., Vega, K., Chung, A., Villena, A., Góñez, C., & Castillo, S. (2002). Effect of *Lepidium meyenii* (MACA) on sexual desire and its absent relationship with serum testosterone levels in adult healthy men. *Andrologia, 34*(6), 367–372. https://doi.org/10.1046/j.1439-0272.2002.00519.x

27. Beharry, S., & Heinrich, M. (2018). Is the hype around the reproductive health claims of maca (*Lepidium meyenii* Walp.) justified? *Journal of Ethnopharmacology, 211,* 126–170. https://doi.org/10.1016/j.jep.2017.08.003

28. Zenico, T., Cicero, A. F. G., Valmorri, L., Mercuriali, M., & Bercovich, E. (2009). Subjective effects of *Lepidium meyenii* (Maca) extract on well-being and sexual performances in patients with mild erectile dysfunction: A randomised, double-blind clinical trial. *Andrologia, 41*(2), 95–99.

29. Gonzales, G. F., Córdova, A., Gonzales, C., Chung, A., Vega, K., & Villena, A. (2001). Improved sperm count after administration of *Lepidium meyenii* (Maca) in adult men. *Asian Journal of Andrology, 3*(4), 3301–3304.

30. Melnikovova, I., Fait, T., Kolarova, M., Fernandez, E. C., & Milella, L. (2015). Effect of *Lepidium meyenii* Walp. on semen parameters and serum hormone levels in healthy adult men: A double-blind, randomized, placebo-controlled pilot study. *Evidence-Based Complementary and Alternative Medicine, 2015,* Article ID 324369. https://doi.org/10.1155/2015/324369

31. Ny, V., Houška, M., Pavela, R., & Tříska, J. (2021). Potential benefits of incorporating *Astragalus membranaceus* into the diet of people undergoing disease treatment: An overview. *Journal of Functional Foods, 77,* 104339. https://doi.org/10.1016/j.jff.2020.104339

32. Sheik, A., Kim, K., Varaprasad, G. L., Lee, H., Kim, S., Kim, E., . . . Huh, Y. S. (2021). The anti-cancerous activity of adaptogenic herb *Astragalus membranaceus. Phytomedicine, 91,* 153698. https://doi.org/10.1016/j.phymed.2021.153698

33. Hong, C. Y., Ku, J., & Wu, P. (1992). *Astragalus membranaceus* stimulates human sperm motility *in vitro. American Journal of Chinese Medicine, 20*(03n04), 289–294. https://doi.org/10.1142/S0192415X92000308

34. Liu, J., Liang, P., Yin, C., Wang, T., Li, H., Li, Y., & Ye, Z. (2004). Effects of several Chinese herbal aqueous extracts on human sperm motility in vitro. *Andrologia, 36*(2), 78–83. https://doi.org/10.1111/j.1439-0272.2004.00607.x

35. Kim, W., Chang, M. S., & Park, S. K. (2016). *Astragalus membranaceus* augment sperm parameters in male mice associated with cAMP-responsive element modulator and activator of CREM in testis. *Journal of Traditional and Complementary Medicine, 6*(3), 294–298. https://doi.org/10.1016/j.jtcme.2015.10.002

36. Hosseini, J., Mardi Mamaghani, A., Hosseinifar, H., Sadighi Gilani, M. A., Dadkhah, F., & Sepidarkish, M. (2016). The influence of ginger (*Zingiber officinale*) on human sperm quality and DNA fragmentation: A double-blind randomized clinical trial. *International Journal of Reproductive Biomedicine, 14*(8), 533–540.

37. Mares, A. K., Abid, W., & Najam, W. S. (2012). The effect of ginger on semen parameters and serum FSH, LH & testosterone of infertile men. *Medical Journal of Tikrit University, 18*(2), 322–329.

CHAPTER 9

1. Domar, A. D., Smith, K., Conboy, L., Iannone, M., & Alper, M. (2010). A prospective investigation into the reasons why insured United States patients drop out of in vitro fertilization treatment. *Fertility and Sterility, 94*(4), 1457–1459. https://doi.org/10.1016/j.fertnstert.2009.06.020

2. Kainz, K. (2001). The role of the psychologist in the evaluation and treatment of infertility. *Women's Health Issues, 11*(6), 481–485. https://doi.org/10.1016/S1049-3867(01)00129-3

3. Khalesi, Z. B., Beiranvand, S. P., & Bokaie, M. (2019). Efficacy of chamomile in the treatment of premenstrual syndrome: A systematic review. *Journal of Pharmacopuncture, 22*(4), 204. https://doi.org/10.3831/kpi.2019.22.028

4. Amsterdam, J. D., Shults, J., Soeller, I., Mao, J. J., Rockwell, K., & Newberg, A. B. (2012). Chamomile (*Matricaria recutita*) may have anti-depressant activity in anxious depressed humans —An exploratory study. *Alternative Therapies in Health and Medicine, 18*(5), 44.

5. Stansbury, J., Saunders, P., & Winston, D. (2012). Supporting adrenal function with adaptogenic herbs. *Journal of Restorative Medicine, 1*(1), 76–82.

6. Ghazizadeh, J., Sadigh-Eteghad, S., Marx, W., Fakhari, A., Hamedeyazdan, S., Torbati, M., . . . Mirghafourvand, M. (2021). The effects of lemon balm (*Melissa officinalis* L.) on depression and anxiety in clinical trials: A systematic review and meta-analysis. *Phytotherapy Research: PTR, 35*(12), 6690–6705. https://doi.org/10.1002/ptr.7252

7. Leproult, R., & Van Cauter, E. (2010). Role of sleep and sleep loss in hormonal release and metabolism. *Endocrine Development, 17,* 11–21. https://doi.org/10.1159/000262524

8. Kumari, P., Jaiswar, S. P., Shankhwar, P., Deo, S., Ahmad, K., Iqbal, B., & Mahdi, A. A. (2017). Leptin as a predictive marker in unexplained infertility in North Indian population. *Journal of Clinical and Diagnostic Research, 11*(3), QC28–QC31. https://doi.org/10.7860/JCDR/2017/22444.9567

9. Ross, R. E., VanDerwerker, C. J., Saladin, M. E., & Gregory, C. M. (2023). The role of exercise in the treatment of depression: Biological under-pinnings and clinical outcomes. *Molecular Psychiatry, 28*(1), 298–328. https://doi.org/10.1038/s41380-022-01819-w

10. Hakimi, O., & Cameron, L. C. (2017). Effect of exercise on ovulation: A systematic review. *Sports Medicine, 47*, 1555–1567. https://doi.org/10.1007/s40279-016-0669-8

11. Dhawan, V., Kumar, M., Deka, D., Malhotra, N., Dadhwal, V., Singh, N., & Dada, R. (2018). Meditation & yoga: Impact on oxidative DNA damage and dysregulated sperm transcripts in male partners of couples with recurrent preg-nancy loss. *Indian Journal of Medical Research, 148*(Suppl), S134–S139. https://doi.org/10.4103/ijmr.IJMR_1988_17

12. Brotto, L. A., Chivers, M. L., Millman, R. D., & Albert, A. (2016). Mindfulness-based sex therapy improves genital-subjective arousal concordance in women with sexual desire/arousal difficulties. *Archives of Sexual Behavior, 45*(8), 1907–1921. https://doi.org/10.1007/s10508-015-0689-8

CHAPTER 10

1. Chiu, Y. H., Afeiche, M. C., Gaskins, A. J., Williams, P. L., Petrozza, J. C., Tanrikut, C., . . . Chavarro, J. E. (2015). Fruit and vegetable intake and their pesticide residues in relation to semen quality among men from a fertility clinic. *Human Reproduction, 30*(6), 1342–1351. https://doi.org/10.1093/humrep/dev064

2. Chiu, Y. H., Williams, P. L., Gillman, M. W., Gaskins, A. J., Mínguez-Alarcón, L., Souter, I., . . . EARTH Study Team. (2018). Association between pesticide residue intake from consumption of fruits and vegetables and pregnancy outcomes among women undergoing infertility treatment with assisted reproductive technology. *JAMA Internal Medicine, 178*(1), 17–26. https://doi.org/10.1001/jamainternmed.2017.5038

3. Oates, L., Cohen, M., Braun, L., Schembri, A., & Taskova, R. (2014). Reduction in urinary organophosphate pesticide metabolites in adults after a week-long organic diet. *Environmental Research, 132*, 105–111. https://doi.org/10.1016/j.envres.2014.03.021

4. Li, D. K., Zhou, Z., Miao, M., He, Y., Wang, J., Ferber, J., . . . Yuan, W. (2011). Urine bisphenol-A (BPA) level in relation to semen quality. *Fertility and Sterility, 95*(2), 625–630.e4. https://doi.org/10.1016/j.fertnstert.2010.09.026

5. Knez, J., Kranvogl, R., Breznik, B. P., Vončina, E., & Vlaisavljević, V. (2014). Are urinary bisphenol A levels in men related to semen quality and embryo development after medically assisted reproduc-tion? *Fertility and Sterility, 101*(1), 215–221. https://doi.org/10.1016/j.fertnstert.2013.09.030

6. Thoene, M., Dzika, E., Gonkowski, S., & Wojtkiewicz, J. (2020). Bisphenol S in food causes hormonal and obesogenic effects comparable to or worse than bisphenol A: A literature review. *Nutrients, 12*(2), 532. https://doi.org/10.3390/nu12020532

7. Radke, E. G., Braun, J. M., Meeker, J. D., & Cooper, G. S. (2018). Phthalate exposure and male reproductive outcomes: A systematic review of the human epidemiological evidence. *Environment International, 121*, 764–793. https://doi.org/10.1016/j.envint.2018.07.029

8. Louis, G. M. B., Sundaram, R., Sweeney, A. M., Schisterman, E. F., Maisog, J., & Kannan, K. (2014). Urinary bisphenol A, phthalates, and couple fecun-dity: The Longitudinal Investigation of Fertility and the Environment (LIFE) study. *Fertility and Sterility, 101*(5), 1359–1366.

9. Mesquita, I., Lorigo, M., & Cairrao, E. (2021). Update about the disrupting-effects of phthalates on the human reproductive system. *Molecular Reproduction and Development, 88*(10), 650–672. https://doi.org/10.1002/mrd.23541

10. Braun, J. M., Just, A. C., Williams, P. L., Smith, K. W., Calafat, A .M., & Hauser, R. (2014). Personal care product use and urinary phthalate metabolite and paraben concentrations during pregnancy among women from a fertility clinic. *Journal of Exposure Science & Environmental Epidemiology, 24*(5), 459–466. https://doi.org/10.1038/jes.2013.69

11. Qian, N., Gao, X., Lang, X., Deng, H., Bratu, T. M., Chen, Q., . . . Min, W. (2024). Rapid single-particle chemical imaging of nanoplastics by SRS microscopy. *Proceedings of the National Academy of Sciences, 121*(3), e2300582121. https://doi.org/10.1073/pnas.2300582121

12. Agarwal, A., Desai, N. R., Mahfouz, R., Mouradi, R., Sharma, R., & Sabanegh, E. (2009). Investigating pathophysiologic effects of cell phone radiation on human spermatozoa: Use of a novel *in vitro* model. *Fertility and Sterility, 92*(3), S221–S222. https://doi.org/10.1016/j.fertnstert.2009.07.1527

13. Zilberlicht, A., Wiener-Megnazi, Z., Sheinfeld, Y., Grach, B., Lahav-Baratz, S., & Dirnfeld, M. (2015). Habits of cell phone usage and sperm quality—does it warrant attention? *Reproductive Biomedicine Online*, *31*(3), 421–426. https://doi.org/10.1016/j.rbmo.2015.06.006

14. Zalata, A., El-Samanoudy, A. Z., Shaalan, D., El-Baiomy, Y., & Mostafa, T. (2015). In vitro effect of cell phone radiation on motility, DNA fragmentation and clusterin gene expression in human sperm. *International Journal of Fertility & Sterility*, *9*(1), 129–136. https://doi.org/10.22074/ijfs.2015.4217

15. See note 13.

16. See note 13.

17. Avendano, C., Mata, A., Sanchez Sarmiento, C. A., & Doncel, G. F. (2012). Use of laptop computers connected to internet through Wi-Fi decreases human sperm motility and increases sperm DNA fragmentation. *Fertility and Sterility*, *97*, 39–45. https://doi.org/10.1016/j.fertnstert.2011.10.012

18. Tommasi, S., Blumenfeld, H., & Besaratinia, A. (2023). Vaping dose, device type, and e-liquid flavor are determinants of DNA damage in electronic cigarette users. *Nicotine and Tobacco Research*, *25*(6), 1145–1154. https://doi.org/10.1093/ntr/ntad003

CHAPTER 11

1. The Rotterdam ESHRE/ASRM-Sponsored PCOS Consensus Workshop Group. (2004). Revised 2003 consensus on diagnostic criteria and long-term health risks related to polycystic ovary syndrome. *Fertility and Sterility*, *81*(1), 19–25. https://doi.org/10.1016/j.fertnstert.2003.10.004

2. Stepto, N. K., Cassar, S., Joham, A. E., Hutchison, S. K., Harrison, C. L., Goldstein, R. F., & Teede, H. J. (2013). Women with polycystic ovary syndrome have intrinsic insulin resistance on euglycaemic–hyperinsulinaemic clamp. *Human Reproduction*, *28*(3), 777–784.

3. Gibson-Helm, M., Teede, H., Dunaif, A., & Dokras, A. (2017). Delayed diagnosis and a lack of information associated with dissatisfaction in women with polycystic ovary syndrome. *The Journal of Clinical Endocrinology and Metabolism*, *102*(2), 604–612. https://doi.org/10.1210/jc.2016-2963

4. Zhang, X., Zheng, Y., Guo, Y., & Lai, Z. (2019). The effect of low carbohydrate diet on polycystic ovary syndrome: A meta-analysis of randomized controlled trials. *International Journal of Endocrinology, 2019*, 4386401. https://doi.org/10.1155/2019/4386401

5. Patten, R. K., McIlvenna, L. C., Levinger, I., Garnham, A. P., Shorakae, S., Parker, A. G., . . . Stepto, N. K. (2022). High-intensity training elicits greater improvements in cardio-metabolic and reproductive outcomes than moderate-intensity training in women with polycystic ovary syndrome: A randomized clinical trial. *Human Reproduction (Oxford, England)*, *37*(5), 1018–1029. https://doi.org/10.1093/humrep/deac047

6. Srnovršnik, T., Virant-Klun, I., & Pinter, B. (2023). Polycystic ovary syndrome and endocrine disruptors (bisphenols, parabens, and triclosan)—A systematic review. *Life (Basel, Switzerland), 13*(1), 138. https://doi.org/10.3390/life13010138

7. Greff, D., Juhász, A. E., Váncsa, S., Váradi, A., Sipos, Z., Szinte, J., . . . Horváth, E. M. (2023). Inositol is an effective and safe treatment in polycystic ovary syndrome: A systematic review and meta-analysis of randomized controlled trials. *Reproductive Biology and Endocrinology: RB&E, 21*(1), 10. https://doi.org/10.1186/s12958-023-01055-z

8. Thakker, D., Raval, A., Patel, I., & Walia, R. (2015). N-acetylcysteine for polycystic ovary syndrome: A systematic review and meta-analysis of randomized controlled clinical trials. *Obstetrics and Gynecology International, 2015*, 817849. https://doi.org/10.1155/2015/817849

9. Spinedi, E., & Cardinali, D. P. (2018). The polycystic ovary syndrome and the metabolic syndrome: A possible chronobiotic-cytoprotective adjuvant therapy. *International Journal of Endocrinology, 2018*, e1349868. https://doi.org/10.1155/2018/1349868

10. Pacchiarotti, A., Carlomagno, G., Antonini, G., & Pacchiarotti, A. (2016). Effect of myo-inositol and melatonin versus myo-inositol, in a randomized controlled trial, for improving in vitro fertilization of patients with polycystic ovarian syndrome. *Gynecological Endocrinology, 32*(1), 69–73. https://doi.org/10.3109/09513590.2015.1101444

11. Kort, D. H., Sullivan, C., Kostolias, A., DePinho, J. C., & Lobo, R. A. (2013). Cinnamon supplementation improves menstrual cyclicity in women with polycystic ovary syndrome. *Fertility and Sterility, 100*(3), S349. https://doi.org/10.1016/j.fertnstert.2013.07.814

12. Wang, J. G., Anderson, R. A., Graham, G. M. III, Chu, M. C., Sauer, M. V., Guarnaccia, M. M., & Lobo, R. A. (2007). The effect of cinnamon extract on insulin resistance parameters in polycystic ovary syndrome: A pilot study. *Fertility and Sterility, 88*(1), 240–243. https://doi.org/10.1016/j.fertnstert.2006.11.082

13. Dastgheib, M., Barati-Boldaji, R., Bahrampour, N., Taheri, R., Borghei, M., Amooee, S., . . . Mazloomi, S. M. (2022). A comparison of the effects of cinnamon, ginger, and metformin consumption on metabolic health, anthropometric indices, and sexual hormone levels in women with poly cystic ovary syndrome: A randomized double-blinded placebo-controlled clinical trial. *Frontiers in Nutrition, 9*, 1071515. https://doi .org/10.3389/fnut.2022.1071515

14. See note 13.

15. Grant, P. (2010). Spearmint herbal tea has significant anti-androgen effects in polycystic ovarian syndrome. A randomized controlled trial. *Phytotherapy Research: An International Journal Devoted to Pharmacological and Toxicological Evaluation of Natural Product Derivatives, 24*(2), 186–188. https://doi.org/10.1002/ptr.2900

16. Takahashi, K., & Kitao, M. (1994). Effect of TJ-68 (*Shakuyaku-kanzo-to*) on polycystic ovarian disease. *International Journal of Fertility and Menopausal Studies, 39*(2), 69–76.

17. Yaginuma, T., Izumi, R., Yasui, H., Arai, T., & Kawabata, M. (1982). Effect of traditional herbal medicine on serum testosterone levels and its induction of regular ovulation in hyperandrogenic and oligomenorrheic women (author's transl). *Nihon Sanka Fujinka Gakkai Zasshi, 34*(7), 939–944.

18. Liu, H., Zeng, L., Yang, K., & Zhang, G. (2016). A network pharmacology approach to explore the pharmacological mechanism of xiaoyao powder on anovulatory infertility. *Evidence-Based Complementary and Alternative Medicine, 2016*, e2960372. https://doi.org/10.1155/2016/2960372

19. Nahata, A., & Dixit, V. K. (2014). Evaluation of 5a-reductase inhibitory activity of certain herbs useful as antiandrogens. *Andrologia, 46*(6), 592–601. https://doi.org/10.1111/and.12115

20. Shahin, A. Y., & Mohammed, S. A. (2014). Adding the phytoestrogen *Cimicifugae racemosae* to clomiphene induction cycles with timed intercourse in polycystic ovary syndrome improves cycle outcomes and pregnancy rates—a randomized trial. *Gynecological Endocrinology, 30*(7), 505–510. https://doi.org/10.3109/09513590.2014.895983

21. Shahin, A. Y., Ismail, A. M., Zahran, K. M., & Makhlouf, A. M. (2008). Adding phytoestrogens to clomiphene induction in unexplained infertility patients—A randomized trial. *Reproductive Biomedicine Online, 16*(4), 580–588. https://doi .org/10.1016/s1472-6483(10)60465-8

22. Feyzollahi, Z., Mohseni Kouchesfehani, H., Jalali, H., Eslimi-Esfahani, D., & Sheikh Hosseini, A. (2021). Effect of *Vitex agnus-castus* ethanolic extract on hypothalamic KISS-1 gene expression in a rat model of polycystic ovary syndrome. *Avicenna Journal of Phytomedicine, 11*(3), 292–301.

23. Fraison, E., Crawford, G., Casper, G., Harris, V., & Ledger, W. (2019). Pregnancy following diagnosis of premature ovarian insufficiency: A systematic review. *Reproductive Biomedicine Online, 39*(3), 467–476.

24. Seidlova-Wuttke, D., & Wuttke, W. (2017). The premenstrual syndrome, premenstrual mastodynia, fibrocystic mastopathy and infertility have often common roots: Effects of extracts of chasteberry (*Vitex agnus castus*) as a solution. *Clinical Phytoscience, 3*, 1–11.

25. Khan, K. N., Fujishita, A., Hiraki, K., Kitajima, M., Nakashima, M., Fushiki, S., & Kitawaki, J. (2018). Bacterial contamination hypothesis: a new concept in endometriosis. *Reproductive Medicine and Biology, 17*(2), 125-133. https://doi .org/10.1002/rmb2.12083

26. Daily, J. W., Zhang, X., Kim, D. S., & Park, S. (2015). Efficacy of ginger for alleviating the symptoms of primary dysmenorrhea: A systematic review and meta-analysis of randomized clinical trials. *Pain Medicine, 16*(12), 2243–2255. https://doi.org/10.1111/pme.12853

27. Marziali, M., Venza, M., Lazzaro, S., Lazzaro, A., Micossi, C., & Stolfi, V. M. (2012). Gluten-free diet: A new strategy for management of painful endometriosis related symptoms? *Minerva Chirurgica, 67*(6), 499–504.

28. Bahat, P. Y., Ayhan, I., Ozdemir, E. U., Inceboz, Ü., & Oral, E. (2022). Dietary supplements for treatment of endometriosis: A review. *Acta Bio Medica: Atenei Parmensis, 93*(1).

29. See note 28.

Index

Page numbers in *italics* indicate illustrations; numbers in **bold** indicate charts.